CARDIOPULMONARY BYPASS:

Current Concepts and Controversies

A Society of Cardiovascular Anesthesiologists Monograph

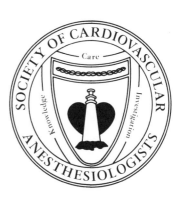

Edited by

John H. Tinker, M.D.

Professor and Head,
Department of Anesthesia,
University of Iowa College of Medicine,
Iowa City, Iowa

1989
W. B. SAUNDERS COMPANY
Harcourt Brace Jovanovich, Inc.
Philadelphia, London, Toronto, Montreal, Sydney, Tokyo

W. B. SAUNDERS COMPANY
Harcourt Brace Jovanovich, Inc.

The Curtis Center
Independence Square West
Philadelphia, PA 19106

RD598
C3538
1989

Library of Congress Cataloging-in-Publication Data

Cardiopulmonary bypass: current concepts and
  controversies / edited by John H. Tinker.
    p. cm—(A Society of Cardiovascular Anesthesiologists
    monograph)

1. Cardiopulmonary bypass.   I. Tinker, John H.
   (John Heath) 1941–   .   II. Series.   [DNLM: 1.
   Cardiopulmonary Bypass.   WG 168 C2655]

RD598.C3538   617'.412059—dc19

DNLM/DLC for Library of Congress   CIP

ISBN 0–7216–8831–4   88–39064

Acquisition Editor: Lisette Bralow

Manuscript Editor: Barbara Hodgson

Production Manager: Frank Polizzano

Indexer: Diana Witt

CARDIOPULMONARY BYPASS: Current Concepts and Controversies
                                    ISBN   0–7216–8831–4

Printed in the United States of America

Last digit is the print number: 9   8   7   6   5   4   3   2   1

Publication Committee of the
Society of Cardiovascular Anesthesiologists

The Society does not endorse the contents of the monograph as policy or as a reflection of the opinion of the members and officers. The monograph does reflect the considered views of each author and, as such, is a worthwhile contribution to the education of the Society membership.

CONTRIBUTORS

NARDA CROUGHWELL, C.R.N.A.

Research Coordinator, Division of Cardiothoracic Anesthesia, and Staff Nurse Anesthetist, Department of Anesthesiology, Heart Center, Duke University Medical Center, Durham, North Carolina.

Anesthesia During Cardiopulmonary Bypass: Does it Matter?

NORIG ELLISON, M.D.

Professor of Anesthesia, Department of Anesthesia, Hospital of the University of Pennsylvania, Philadelphia, Pennsylvania.

Hemostasis During Cardiopulmonary Bypass

ANN V. GOVIER, M.D.

Staff Anesthesiologist, Department of Cardio-Thoracic Anesthesia, The Cleveland Clinic Foundation, Cleveland, Ohio.

Central Nervous System Complications after Cardiopulmonary Bypass

WILLIAM J. GREELEY, M.D.

Assistant Professor of Anesthesiology and Assistant Professor of Pediatrics, Duke University Medical Center, Durham, North Carolina.

Anesthesia During Cardiopulmonary Bypass: Does it Matter?

DOLLY D. HANSEN, M.D.

Assistant Professor of Anaesthesia (Pediatrics), Harvard Medical School. Senior Associate in Anesthesia, Boston Children's Hospital, Boston, Massachusetts.

Temperature and Blood Gases: The Clinical Dilemma of Acid–Base Management for Hypothermic Cardiopulmonary Bypass

PAUL R. HICKEY, M.D.

Associate Professor of Anaesthesia, Harvard Medical School. Senior Associate in Anesthesia, Boston Children's Hospital, Boston, Massachusetts.

Temperature and Blood Gases: The Clinical Dilemma of Acid–Base Management for Hypothermic Cardiopulmonary Bypass

JAMES R. JACOBS, Ph.D.
Assistant Professor of Anesthesia and Assistant Professor of Biomedical Engineering, Duke University Medical Center, Durham, North Carolina.
Anesthesia During Cardiopulmonary Bypass: Does it Matter?

DAVID R. JOBES, M.D.
Associate Professor of Anesthesia, Department of Anesthesia, Hospital of the University of Pennsylvania, Philadelphia, Pennsylvania.
Hemostasis During Cardiopulmonary Bypass

JAMES K. KIRKLIN, M.D.
Professor of Surgery, Division of Cardiothoracic Surgery, and Director of Cardiac Transplantation, University of Alabama, Birmingham, Alabama.
The Postperfusion Syndrome: Inflammation and the Damaging Effects of Cardiopulmonary Bypass

JOHN R. MOYERS, M.D.
Associate Professor, Department of Anesthesia, University of Iowa College of Medicine. Chief, Cardiovascular Anesthesia, University of Iowa Hospitals and Clinics, Iowa City, Iowa.
Emergence from Cardiopulmonary Bypass: Controversies about Physiology and Pharmacology

J. G. REVES, M.D.
Professor of Anesthesiology and Director of the Heart Center, Duke University Medical Center, Durham, North Carolina.
Anesthesia During Cardiopulmonary Bypass: Does it Matter?

IAN R. THOMSON, M.D.
Associate Professor, University of Manitoba. Section Head, Cardiovascular Anesthesia, St. Boniface General Hospital, Winnipeg, Manitoba.
The Influence of Cardiopulmonary Bypass on Cerebral Physiology and Function

JOHN H. TINKER, M.D.
Professor and Head, Department of Anesthesia, University of Iowa College of Medicine, Iowa City, Iowa.
Emergence from Cardiopulmonary Bypass: Controversies about Physiology and Pharmacology

PREFACE

Cardiopulmonary bypass was first successful in 1953. After 36 years it might be assumed that techniques and management would be well standardized. My travels to cardiac operating rooms around the United States, Canada, and elsewhere have convinced me that such is not the case. Not too long ago I observed a situation in which the perfusionist was trying to maintain mean arterial pressure below 60 mm Hg, whereas the anesthesiologist wanted the pressure considerably higher. The latter individual would increase his phenylephrine infusion, whereupon, after a few minutes, the perfusionist, noting that the arterial pressure had crept upward, would decrease the pump flow! This went on for a considerable period, not because there was the slightest animosity between the anesthesiologist and the perfusionist, but simply because they were not in the habit of communicating. Another time, in a different university teaching hospital, I observed the perfusionist administering 5-mg boluses of chlorpromazine whenever the arterial pressure would increase above 50 mm Hg. Over about 50 minutes the perfusionist gave a total of 25 mg of Thorazine to the patient. I told the anesthesiologist afterward about this, and was greeted by disbelief!

At this writing there are no accurate national data, but based on informal polls held at meetings, conversations with officials from perfusionist organizations, and so on, I would estimate that at least half of the cardiopulmonary bypass administered in the United States and Canada is now being done using the "alpha-stat" method of acid–base management. This represents a change from virtually all bypass formerly using "pH-stat" management in the early 1980s. Further, the change to alpha-stat management seems to have occurred *before* there was substantial literature evidence to warrant it. To be sure, there was knowledge about how poikilothermic animals control their acid–base balance, and some evidence that human peripheral tissues behave similarly when they become hypothermic. Nonetheless, perfusionists (with the tacit approval of surgeons and anesthesiologists—if they indeed understood what was happening) simply began dropping $Paco_2$ (actual, corrected for temperature) into the low 20s in humans. Subsequent to the start of that, evidence from several studies shows that there is overall "matching" at least of lowered cerebral blood flow and cerebral oxygen demand. No studies yet, in animals or humans, have shown that *regional* cerebral flow and demand are just as well matched, especially when there is vascular disease.

We still reverse heparin with protamine. Heparin is given in widely varying amounts. Reversal is by protocol in some centers, by clotting studies in others. Clotting studies include test tubes with brown sand in them and/or other test tubes with salmon sperm extract in them. Various numbers that are generated by the automated machines that perform these tests are relied on to make important clinical decisions—decision points that differ considerably between institutions.

Numerous other areas of controversy exist; for example, pump flows range from 1.0 to 2.5 $1 \cdot min^{-1} \cdot m^{-2}$. Methods of producing anesthesia vary widely. Whether or not anesthesia is necessary during bypass is controversial. Bypass clearly is increasingly detrimental to the patient's internal homeostasis—but only recently have we begun to make much sense out of the many isolated findings about complement activation, the stress response, blood flow distribution, and the like.

Emergence from bypass is a time of anxiety for everyone in the cardiac operating room. Inotropes, vasodilators, intra-aortic balloon pumps, left ventricular assist devices are all difficult to decide on, and controversy surrounds their various uses, benefits, and drawbacks.

The impetus for this monograph grew from several workshops on cardiopulmonary bypass held by the Society of Cardiovascular Anesthesiologists. These workshops have convinced many of us that there is now strong interest, not just among anesthesiologists, but also among perfusionists and surgeons, in trying to understand bypass physiology, pathophysiology, and pharmacology. Neurologic and neuropsychiatric dysfunction remain a major risk after bypass. Perhaps this area, more than any other single motive, drives us all to seek better understanding of bypass.

This book contains state-of-the-art reviews of the controversial areas mentioned above. Each review was written by experts who gave more than generously of immensely valuable time. I salute and profoundly thank all the contributors. I think that this book will add considerably to our understanding of cardiopulmonary bypass. It wouldn't surprise me if the next "generation" of cardiac anesthesiologists might just find in it a germ or two of an idea to further our knowledge. I enjoyed reading and editing and learning from the experts as this book took shape.

JOHN H. TINKER, M.D.
Iowa City, Iowa

CONTENTS

CHAPTER

1 TEMPERATURE AND BLOOD GASES: The Clinical
Dilemma of Acid–Base Management for
Hypothermic Cardiopulmonary Bypass 1
Paul R. Hickey and Dolly D. Hansen

CHAPTER

2 THE INFLUENCE OF CARDIOPULMONARY
BYPASS ON CEREBRAL PHYSIOLOGY
AND FUNCTION 21
Ian R. Thomson

CHAPTER

3 CENTRAL NERVOUS SYSTEM COMPLICATIONS
AFTER CARDIOPULMONARY BYPASS 41
Ann V. Govier

CHAPTER

4 ANESTHESIA DURING CARDIOPULMONARY
BYPASS: Does it Matter? 69
J. G. Reves, Narda Croughwell, James R. Jacobs,
and William Greeley

CHAPTER

5 HEMOSTASIS DURING CARDIOPULMONARY
BYPASS 99
Norig Ellison and David R. Jobes

CHAPTER

6 EMERGENCE FROM CARDIOPULMONARY
BYPASS: Controversies about Physiology and
Pharmacology 109
John R. Moyers and John H. Tinker

CHAPTER

7   THE POSTPERFUSION SYNDROME: Inflammation
      and the Damaging Effects of Cardiopulmonary
      Bypass 131
      James K. Kirklin

INDEX   147

TEMPERATURE AND BLOOD GASES: The Clinical Dilemma of Acid–Base Management for Hypothermic Cardiopulmonary Bypass

PAUL R. HICKEY and DOLLY D. HANSEN

Despite more than 30 years of clinical experience with hypothermic cardiopulmonary bypass (CPB), the controversy over temperature correction of blood gases remains unresolved. The lack of resolution stems in part from failure to understand the issues. Actually, whether or not to use temperature correction of arterial blood gases is only the "tip of the iceberg." The larger and only really important question concerns optimal acid–base management for hypothermia during CPB.

Corrected and uncorrected arterial blood gases are simply different scales, somewhat like different temperature scales. The same relative acid–base status gives different numbers depending on which technique is used because each is referenced differently and conversion factors must be used for each "scale." Similarly, when moving between centigrade and Fahrenheit temperature measurements, conversion factors must be used between the different scales. Although use of uncorrected and corrected blood gases simplifies implementation, respectively, of "alpha-stat" and "pH-stat" acid–base regulation, the important physiologic issue is the amount of H^+ *relative* to OH^- present in blood (or intracellularly), not the absolute amount of H^+ present. If the clinical objective is electrochemical neutrality, equally "excess" amounts of H^+ are present in blood at 25° C whether *uncorrected* pH is 7.3 or *corrected* pH is 7.5. Acid–base management can be implemented using either blood gas "scale" once acid–base requirements are determined and understood.

That this larger question of what are proper hypothermic acid–base

1

requirements remains after 30 years suggests that either acid–base management is not particularly critical for tissue preservation during hypothermic bypass, or that other factors influence tissue preservation and thus blur critical effects of acid–base regulation. It is also possible that many more gross problems of bypass, unsolved until recent years, obscured subtle differences in outcome resulting from acid–base management. Substantial dissimilarities that exist in myocardial and/or cerebral outcome resulting from the two greatly different types of acid–base management, alpha- or pH-stat, should be apparent by now. Thus the question under consideration is either trivial, of primarily academic interest, or is subtler and/or more complex than is currently detectable.

There are three ways to measure blood gases: (1) with the measuring apparatus itself at body temperature; (2) with blood warmed anaerobically (hopefully) and measured in the analyzer at 37° C and then "corrected" back to body temperature using calculations or nomograms; and (3) with raw "uncorrected" values obtained from anaerobically warmed blood. The first technique was not used clinically until recently, with the advent of the new optical fluorescence bypass methodology (the validity of which is not yet fully established). The first two values, those actually made at body temperature and those "corrected" to body temperature, are roughly equivalent except that values measured at body temperature are generally more accurate than those corrected back to body temperature. Throughout the following discussion, distinctions between different ways of measuring and referencing arterial blood gases must be kept in mind.

HISTORICAL BACKGROUND

Regulation Using pH-stat

Traditionally, physicians have been trained to recognize arterial pH of about 7.40 and Pa_{CO_2} of 40 as "normal," indicative of neutral acid–base balance. Physicians are rarely taught *why* these values are important, and until relatively recently "normal" values have not been questioned. Only in the past decade have physicians begun to recognize that these traditional acid–base concepts of normality may not apply to hypothermic people, although comparative physiologists have long known that traditional concepts apply only to tissues at 37° C. Physiologists recognized various aspects of this problem as early as 1919[1]; alterations of O_2, CO_2, and pH equilibria with anaerobic cooling of blood were recognized before 1950.[2] However, these considerations were of little practical import to physicians until development of hypothermic CPB presented the dilemma of proper acid–base management during hypothermia.

Traditional concepts of acid–base regulation, coupled with Severinghaus' publication of detailed and accurate nomograms for temperature changes in arterial blood gases in 1959,[3, 4] led to uncritical use of normal *corrected* values of arterial pH and $Paco_2$ (7.4 and 40 mm Hg) during the first two decades of hypothermic bypass. Because CO_2 solubility increases with temperature, total body CO_2 stores must be increased during cooling to maintain these "normal" corrected values. Five per cent CO_2 was added to oxygenator gas flows to maintain corrected pH 7.4 and $Paco_2$ 40 mm Hg. Additional CO_2 was necessary partly because of decreased CO_2 production with cooling and partly because higher gas flows required by early oxygenators (and/or preferred by perfusionists) tended to remove large amounts of CO_2. Lack of knowledge about hypothermic cerebral autoregulation and the all-too-common occurrence of severe neurologic complications with early hypothermic bypass further reinforced the practice of adding CO_2, which was presumed to maintain cerebral vasodilation and "normal" levels of cerebral blood flow.

This type of hypothermic acid–base regulation has been termed "pH-stat" because *corrected* (i.e., actual) pH and $Paco_2$ are kept constant. Nomograms for temperature correction of arterial blood gases are required to implement this mode of regulation. Accuracy of these nomograms is somewhat limited because hematocrit, protein concentration, and other factors frequently are changed substantially during CPB using hemodilution.

Regulation Using Alpha-stat

Investigations by comparative physiologists into acid–base regulation of ectothermic or poikilothermic animals with varying body temperatures laid the foundation for a better understanding of acid–base regulation during hypothermia.[5–7] Starting in the 1960s, Rahn and Reeves[8–13] built on early work and developed a unified concept of acid–base regulation that appeared to apply to fish, reptiles, and amphibians whose body temperatures varied over wide ranges (Fig. 1–1). This unified concept is based on maintenance of *intracellular electrochemical neutrality* at all temperatures and *seems* to apply to normothermic and hypothermic humans.[7] By keeping total CO_2 stores constant, net protein charge states (termed "alpha") are kept constant as temperature changes so that this regulation is termed "alpha-stat." The "alpha" refers to the most important charged species, the alpha imidazole ring on the histidine amino acid moiety in various proteins. Alpha-stat regulation is most easily implemented clinically by simply maintaining normal *uncorrected* levels of pH_a and $Paco_2$ at 7.4 and 40 mm Hg, respectively. Thus no nomograms are required to implement this type of regulation.

In the early 1980s the alpha-stat approach to acid–base management

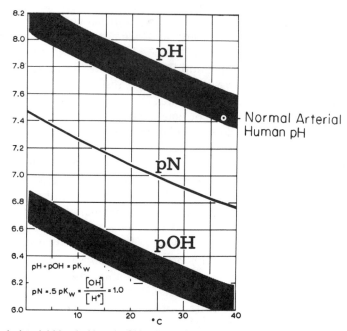

Figure 1–1. Arterial blood pH and pOH values of various cold-blooded vertebrates at various body temperatures. These values parallel the chemical neutrality of water (pN). The numbers of H^+ and OH^- are equal at pN. (Adapted with permission from Rahn H: Body temperature and acid–base regulation. Pneumonologie 151:87, 1974.)

appeared in anesthetic, cardiac surgical, and perfusion literature and began to be applied widely to hypothermic patients during CPB because of compelling theoretical arguments in its favor.[14–18] This occurred despite lack of substantial clinical outcome studies or other evidence, and no randomized trials. Subsequently, alpha-stat has become a predominant mode of hypothermic acid–base management among many centers in the United States and abroad. It is currently estimated that half of CPB is managed each way. Arguments for using alpha-stat are largely theoretical; few clinical data are available to prove superiority of alpha-stat over pH-stat regulation. Indeed, recent experimental data, outlined below, suggest that the problem of hypothermic acid–base balance is considerably more complex than a simple choice between alpha-stat and pH-stat management.

THEORETICAL BASIS AND RATIONALE FOR ALPHA-STAT ACID–BASE REGULATION

Normal protein structure and function, particularly enzyme function, depends on a constant and usually neutral electrochemical environment because electrochemical charge states and binding are largely responsible for maintaining normal protein conformational structure. Acid–base regulatory systems provide, in most cases, a neutral intracellular milieu in which hydrogen ions (H^+) and hydroxyl ions (OH^-) are equal in number, thus maintaining a constant ratio, $H^+/OH^- = 1$. Traditional concepts of acid–base regulation have suggested, wrongly, that normality is defined by pH (i.e., the *number* of hydrogen ions) rather than by the *ratio* between H^+ and OH^-.

The term pH defines the actual number of hydrogen ions in solution (although we are saddled with the handicap that Sorensen thought it would be a good idea to use the negative log of the H^+ concentration). In aqueous solutions such as cells and blood the primary source of hydrogen is water; the dissociation constant of water, pK_w, largely controls pH. Long ignored was the fact that pK_w *increases* as temperature decreases, so that hydrogen ion number decreases and pH, the negative log, *increases* as aqueous solutions cool. The pH of electrochemical neutrality, pN, increases nonlinearly along with pK_w because $pN = 0.5 \, pK_w$ (Fig. 1–1). In neutral, cooling aqueous solutions, hydroxyl ions, which also are controlled by pK_w, decrease in tandem with H^+. This maintains a constant H^+-OH^- ratio. Thus pH of electrochemical neutrality in aqueous solutions changes with temperature.

Importance of Intracellular Neutrality for Normal Cell Function

Protein structure and function, optimal reaction rates of important enzyme systems, and intracellular concentrations of critical metabolic intermediates are all critically dependent on constant, neutral intracellular environments. This is an extension of Claude Bernard's concept of the "milieu interieur." The appropriate pH for a given temperature that maintains a normal H^+-OH^- ratio (i.e., neutrality) preserves normal charged ionic states of cytosolic intermediary metabolites and maintains active sites of critical enzymes. Davis[19] surveyed ionization constants (pK_a) of hundreds of water-soluble biosynthetic intermediates and found that these fleeting intermediates are completely ionized only in the region of electrochemical neutrality at various temperatures. Intracellular accumulation of hydrogen ions from any cause moves intracellular pH (pH_i) out of the neutral zone for that temperature and metabolites lose their charged state, becoming un-ionized. These uncharged, now lipophilic molecules can freely diffuse down concentration gradients across lipid cellular membranes, depleting intracellular concentrations. Depleted intracellular concentrations of these important metabolic intermediates can theoretically retard generation of high-energy phosphates. In contrast, at neutral pH_i for any given temperature, metabolic intermediates that are ionized have little tendency to cross lipid membranes.

Accumulation of excess hydrogen ions decreases pH_i below neutrality and may poison various active sites of intracellular enzymes critical for generation of high-energy phosphates. Most enzymes are dependent on optimal pH for maximum function. This optimal pH of most enzymes changes with temperature in tandem with pN, the neutral pH of water.[20] This seems particularly true for enzymes involved in generation of high-energy phosphates.[20] Thus a pH_i lower than pN at any tissue temperature may lead to loss of critical metabolic intermediates, decreasing substrate levels, and lower levels of critical enzyme function.

Electrochemical neutrality in cells also preserves the Donnan equilibrium across cellular membranes, maintaining normal intracellular anion concentration and water content.[9] Thus preservation of appropriately neutral pH_i during hypothermia, by maintaining electrochemical neutrality, is linked to many aspects of cellular function and viability: preservation of high-energy phosphates, concentrations of metabolites, structure of proteins, function of enzymes, ion concentrations, and cell volumes. It must be added that these arguments, though compelling, are biochemical and theoretical and are not yet clinically tested.

Intracellular and Extracellular Buffering of Neutral pH

Keeping a constant intracellular H^+-OH^- at 37° C requires buffering systems that maintain intracellular pH_e around 6.8 to 6.9. This is facilitated by maintaining arterial blood pH at about 7.4 for "neutrality." The pH of extracellular fluid is usually that of pH_i plus a varying and poorly understood species-specific factor of around 0.6 to 0.8 pH units. Because of log factors involved, although optimal intracellular H^+-OH^- is 1:1, adding in this species-specific factor results in an extracellular (and blood) pH of about 7.4, providing an extracellular H^+-OH^- of around 1:16. This means that blood and extracellular fluid are normally relatively alkaline at "neutral" blood pH. This normal extracellular-to-intracellular hydrogen ion gradient allows for unloading of acidic products of cellular metabolism, including CO_2, to extracellular space and blood. It is essential to understand at this point that neutral pH changes with temperature; maintenance of neutral intracellular H^+-OH^- of 1:1 at 20° C requires pH_i of 7.1. Maintenance of normal relative extracellular and blood alkalinity with H^+-OH^- of 1:16, therefore, requires blood pH of 7.7, the "neutral" blood pH at this temperature.

In blood, and particularly inside cells, the CO_2–bicarbonate buffer system is only a small part of total buffering capacity responsible for maintaining pN intracellularly and a pH = pN + 0.6 pH units in blood. The great majority of intracellular and extracellular buffering is provided by protein buffers. By far the most important and dominant protein buffer is the imidazole R-group of the amino acid histidine, which is abundant in most proteins.[9] As temperature drops, this imidazole protein buffer changes its pK_a in parallel with pN of water. Because of this parallelism, pH_i (and, at a higher level, blood pH) increases along the same slope as pH when temperature falls *as long as total CO_2 stores remain unchanged*. If this occurs, the fraction of unprotonated histidine imidazole groups, known as alpha, remains constant but pH changes. This is the essence of alpha-stat acid–base management; the fraction of unprotonated imidazole groups (protein charge) remains constant, total CO_2 remains constant, and pH changes as temperature changes. Constant alpha means that net charge on proteins is protected from change as temperature and pH change. Constant net charge maintains normal protein structure and function as well as other aspects of intracellular homeostasis.

EVIDENCE FOR ALPHA-STAT OR OTHER ACID–BASE REGULATION IN COLD-BLOODED VERTEBRATES AND IN HUMANS

Normal acid–base strategies followed by humans and cold-blooded vertebrates at different environmental temperatures provide considerable insight into questions of optimal acid–base management. Generally, alpha-stat is followed, but lower animals have some specialized adaptations for acid–base management during hypothermia. These comparative physiologic data are used to justify various approaches to acid–base management during hypothermic CPB in humans.

Cold-Blooded Vertebrates

A series of experiments in cold-blooded vertebrates whose body temperatures fluctuate with the environment were done by Rahn and Reeves,[11-13, 21, 22] but the concepts were initially reported by Austin et al. in 1927[6] and Robin in 1962.[7] These observations showed that arterial pH increased and $Paco_2$ decreased precisely as body temperature fell in a variety of animals, including frogs, toads, and turtles. Arterial pH and pOH in these animals are shown in Figure 1–1. These changes in arterial pH with temperature parallel pH changes in chemically neutral water (pN). Intracellular pH (pH_i) of various tissues in cold-blooded animals was measured as a function of body temperature by Malan et al.[23] Intracellular pH of most tissues showed identical changes with temperature that were parallel and virtually identical to the pN of water. Virtual identity of pH_i changes with those of pN of water in a variety of species is strong evidence for alpha-stat theory as it applies to poikilotherms, but whether this applies to humans during hypothermic CPB is unknown.

Air-breathing cold-blooded vertebrates adjust their blood acid–base balance with temperature changes by modifying ventilation as their metabolic rate changes so that total CO_2 remains constant, maintaining constant alpha. They are, in essence, hyperventilating, i.e., decreasing ventilation *less* than the commensurate decrease in CO_2 production caused by the lowered temperature. Water-breathers, in contrast, are dependent on inefficient oxygen extraction from gills and cannot adjust CO_2 by changing ventilation without becoming severely hypoxemic. Instead, they actively transport ions across gill epithelia, taking up and excreting strong basic cations (which is energetically very costly and slow) in order to maintain appropriate pH for alpha-stat.[24] Their changing CO_2 stores resulting from activity and temperature changes cannot easily be regulated because of inefficient modes of gill gas exchange underwater, but still they do appear to maintain constant alpha states as temperatures change.

Thus alpha-stat acid–base regulatory strategy is followed by cold-blooded vertebrates whose tissues must function normally despite wide variations in tissue temperature. Temperature variations in these lower animals are wider in range and may require different compensatory mechanisms in some cases, such as in water-breathers. Water-breathers that function at extremes of hypothermia in cold ocean waters under ice down to 4° C must use still other adaptive mechanisms, such as rapid changes in phospholipid composition of cellular membranes as temperature changes. These adaptations are necessary in order to protect lipid membranes from changes in physical state and to preserve of normal membrane functions at very low temperatures.[25] If these adaptations are elucidated, this may shed some light on several human problems. Ice-water drowning victims, long episodes of deep hypothermic circulatory arrest, and profound clinical hypothermia to less than 10° C all are often associated with poor outcomes. There appears to be a point in these clinical circumstances, both in temperature and time, wherein hypothermia changes from protective to harmful. Clearly much research needs to be done in this fascinating field.

Humans

In human blood cooled in vitro without gas exchange, pH and Pa_{CO_2} changes occur similar to those in cold-blooded vertebrates with changing body temperatures. These changes are demonstrated in a closed syringe of human blood in vitro and have been observed in arterial blood and in body fluids of hypothermic patients on bypass.[2, 26] As temperature decreases, Pa_{CO_2} falls as CO_2 becomes more soluble, but plasma bicarbonate concentration and total CO_2 does not change in human blood when gas exchange is prevented. These Pa_{CO_2} and pH changes with temperature are remarkably constant in human blood over a wide range of both initial acid–base conditions and moderate variations in hematocrit.[8] Rahn has pointed out that arterial blood of a "normothermic" human represents a heterogeneity of pHs, depending on the temperature of various tissues.[10] If pH and Pa_{CO_2} of various tissues of a person exercising in cold are measured (at tissue temperature), then arterial blood ejected from the heart has "normal" values (7.40, 40 mm Hg), but when that same blood arrives at muscle masses exercising at 42° C, the values change to preserve alpha (7.35, 47 mm Hg), since no gas exchange takes place in the arterial tree. Other blood in the same person, cooled to 25° C in transit to skin has quite different values (7.60, 23 mm Hg). The very cold hands of this person at 7° C have still different arterialized blood gas values (7.66, 16 mm Hg). These changes in blood temperature, pH, and P_{CO_2} occur at constant CO_2, since no CO_2 exchange occurs during transit through the arterial tree, so these values of pH and P_{CO_2} are normal physiologic values *for the temperatures at which these tissues are operating.* If arterial blood from any of these tissues is sampled and warmed to 37° C in a clinical blood gas analyzer, all samples would read the same uncorrected values of 7.40 and 40 mm Hg because total CO_2 stores are unchanged (i.e., an alpha-stat system).

By maintaining constant total CO_2, arterial pH is maintained on the alkaline side of intracellular electrochemical neutrality in all tissues regardless of local temperature changes. Presumably, although not yet reported, pH_i in normally functioning human tissues behaves similarly, at slightly more acidotic levels.

This evidence for alpha-stat acid–base regulation in humans illustrates that "normal" arterial pH in functioning human tissues varies depending on tissue temperature; thus 7.4 is normal arterial pH only at 37° C. When exercising in any hypothermic environment, such as running in winter, we are engaging in natural experiments in hypothermia and hyperthermia wherein a spectrum of "normal" arterial pH values exists simultaneously in human tissues functioning at different temperatures.

RELATION BETWEEN INTRACELLULAR AND EXTRACELLULAR pH

Up to this point it has been implicitly assumed that because of similar buffering systems, intracellular and extracellular pH change in parallel but are separated by a fixed gradient so that changes in one will be reflected by similar changes in the other. Intracellular–extracellular pH gradient (pH_i–pH_e) is attributed to active mechanisms in cellular membranes and selective membrane permeability as well as different intracellular buffering capacity, but the arguments above assume that the gradient does not change under various conditions. Further, the assumption is made that the pH_i–pH_e gradients are equal in all tissues. Unfortunately it has become increasingly clear that these assumptions grossly oversimplify matters in critical ways.

Hibernating Mammals

Initially it appeared that small hibernating mammals followed pH-stat rather than alpha-stat regulation during hibernation. Constant blood pH_a and $Paco_2$ values (measured at existing body temperature) are maintained during hibernation; this is pH-stat acid–base regulation.[27] It is equivalent to maintaining corrected pH and $Paco_2$ values of 7.4 and 40 mm Hg in a hypothermic patient on bypass and has been used as an argument for following pH-stat strategy clinically. Hibernating mammals maintain constant corrected blood pH_a and $Paco_2$; therefore, their total CO_2 stores must increase as CO_2 solubility increases with cold. If the previously discussed theory is valid, this should create relative respiratory acidosis because $Paco_2$ should have decreased with temperature. The excess CO_2 would freely diffuse across cell membranes, so pH_i would become acidotic during hibernation in most tissues.

When pH_i is acidotic in diverse metabolic systems, from bacteria to higher organisms, metabolism becomes depressed.[28] This depression of metabolic function indeed occurs in various metabolic systems of hibernators such as muscle glycolysis, norepinephrine-mediated nonshivering thermogenesis mediated by brown fat, and others. It is mediated partly through marked inhibition of normal enzyme function in key metabolic pathways by relatively small decreases in pH_i. Williamson et al.[29] studied effects of induced intracellular acidosis on mammalian cardiac muscle metabolism and showed that glycolytic flux decreased by 71 per cent and lactate-pyruvate ratio increased tenfold when pH_i was decreased from 6.95 to 6.57. This is due largely to inhibition of lactate dehydrogenase and phosphofructokinase activity with decreasing pH_i.

Transition from an acidotic intracellular condition (pH-stat) to alpha-stat condition is marked by activation of metabolic processes. Correspondingly the opposite change (i.e., pH_i decreases of only a few tenths) can result in large decreases in metabolic function.[20] In small hibernating mammals using pH-stat strategy, such alterations in metabolism are very useful for nonfunctioning tissues such as skeletal muscle, gastrointestinal tract, and higher brain centers because acidosis-mediated decreases in cellular metabolism appear to further decrease the already markedly depressed hypothermic cellular metabolism, providing cell death does not supervene.

In tissues that must function during hibernation, such as heart and liver, intracellular acidosis with depression of tissue metabolism associated with pH-stat should be a disadvantage. These active tissues appear to compensate for relative acidosis of pH-stat blood by actively extruding H^+ across their plasma membranes by way of energy-dependent ion exchange, at the additional cost of accumulating intracellular bicarbonate.[27] Thus pH_i of these tissues (heart and liver) is maintained at or near alpha-stat values, at the expense of somewhat greater acidosis in blood and nonfunctioning tissues. Hibernators appear to be able to vary pH_i–pH_e gradient in some tissues, maintaining different types of acid–base regulation in each.

When these mammals go into hibernation, they hypoventilate, accumulate CO_2 stores, and build up a respiratory acidosis. In contrast, on beginning arousal while still very hypothermic, the first overt physiologic process is hyperventilation, which depletes accumulated CO_2 stores, thus raising pH_i so that metabolic activation can begin in previously dormant, acidotic tissues. Subsequently, increases in metabolic rates and heat production result. This reversion to alpha-stat regulation appears to occur before any increase in metabolic rate and increase in body temperature. Thus blood and quiescent tissues of hypothermic hibernating mammals appear to convert to alpha-stat acid–base regulation when tissue function and normal (for temperature) metabolic rates are necessary. In contrast, functioning heart and liver tissues maintain near alpha-stat continuously during hypothermia. These data suggest that alpha-stat control is optimal for *functioning tissues* regardless of temperature. Still unknown are mechanisms whereby cell damage during rather severe intracellular acidosis is avoided and full functional capacity is restored quickly to tissues when CO_2 stores are unloaded and pH rises to alpha-stat levels throughout the body.

Reptiles and Amphibians

Bickler recently found that brain pH_i of lizards stayed constant over an 18° to 35° C temperature range (pH-stat), whereas other tissue compartments, including blood, conformed to alpha-stat models.[30] In another species, pH_i of white muscle, heart, and esophagus also changed little with temperature, corresponding to pH-stat control.[31] In two species of toads, blood pH–temperature relation conformed to alpha-stat–type patterns over temperatures ranging from 10° to 30° C, whereas pH_i in a variety of different muscles showed considerable variation with temperature, but only partially followed alpha-stat mechanisms.[32] Further, other data suggest that intracellular tissue buffering deviates considerably from classic histidine-imidazole alpha-stat buffering.[33] These data point out that intracellular acid–base regulation can be independent of blood regulation and does not always follow alpha-stat, both within and among different groups of animals.

THEORETICAL IMPLICATIONS FOR ACID–BASE
MANAGEMENT DURING HYPOTHERMIC BYPASS IN HUMANS

How, then, should acid–base balance be regulated during hypothermia in humans? Unfortunately there are no data suggesting how local tissue regulation of pH_i similar to that seen in hibernators and others might apply in humans. If such local regulation of pH_i in humans was important, it might make the question of hypothermic acid–base regulation of blood somewhat academic, and in that case, control of blood (and extracellular) pH during bypass would be less critical.

Further, the optimal intracellular state for preservation of human tissues during hypothermia is unknown. Moderate acidosis with depression of hypothermic cellular metabolic activity beyond that caused by hypothermia alone might be optimal, or, alternatively, neutrality with optimal maintenance of enzyme functional capacity and protein structure might be best. This review of comparative physiology shows that in all organisms, humans as well as amphibians, reptiles, and hibernating mammals, most *functioning* tissues maintain their pH_i at or close to alpha-stat requirements as tissue temperatures change. When the organism as a whole must function, blood pH also follows alpha-stat acid–base balance, although specific tissues may regulate pH_i independently.

None of this tells us if acid–base management is critical or, if so, what constitutes optimal management of a patient during hypothermic CPB. Should we attempt to maintain intracellular and blood pH at alpha-stat levels that are clearly best for *normal* tissue function during hypothermia? Alternatively, should we use pH-stat with accumulation of CO_2, relative intracellular acidosis, and depression of normal metabolism and function in the entire body, since perhaps no tissues need to function normally while cold on bypass? Perhaps pH-stat with depression of metabolism would be protective when critical tissues such as heart and brain are subjected, deliberately or accidentally, to ischemia during bypass. On the other hand, this approach exposes critical human tissues to effects of acute acidosis without evidence for specialized membrane mechanisms with which hibernators locally control pH_i in critical tissues. It further assumes that normal function can be restored with rewarming and restoration of neutral pH_i. Unfortunately, relevant data regarding damage to tissues managed with various acid–base strategies are scanty.

EFFECTS OF ACID–BASE REGULATION ON ORGAN
FUNCTION AND PRESERVATION IN HYPOTHERMIC
HUMANS AND ANIMALS

Brain

Anesthesiologists have long had concerns about effects of acid–base regulation on cerebral blood flow during hypothermia. Experimentally, cerebral autoregulation for flow and pressure has been shown to be intact in monkeys on bypass at 20° C, but CO_2 reactivity was not assessed in this study.[34] Govier et al.[35] studied autoregulation of regional cerebral blood flow in hypothermic patients during bypass using alpha-stat management and found intact cerebral autoregulation at temperatures ranging from 21° to 29° C. Cerebral blood flow changed little with pressure or flow but varied significantly with temperature and $Paco_2$. Cerebral CO_2 reactivity was also found to be well preserved in hypothermic patients on bypass by Lundar et al.,[36] particularly at cerebral perfusion pressures greater than 20 mm Hg. Prough et al.[37] reported that response of the cerebral circulation in hypothermic humans to changes in $Paco_2$ from 36 to 53 mm Hg (uncorrected) was well maintained. From this study it is clear that following alpha-stat and maintaining uncorrected $Paco_2$ at 40 mm Hg results in significantly lower cerebral blood flow than when pH-stat is followed and corrected $Paco_2$ is kept around 40 (uncorrected $Paco_2$ is about 55 at this temperature). However, Fox et al.[38] and others have documented large decreases in cerebral metabolic rate in humans during hypothermic bypass. This introduces the question of the appropriate level of cerebral blood flow during hypothermia, since clearly acid–base regulation can alter cerebral flow. Also, though, it says nothing about regional cerebral blood flow, intracerebral steal possibilities, and the like.

Murkin et al.[39] have shown effects of $Paco_2$ on *global* flow-metabolism coupling in human brain during hypothermic (26° C) CPB. When uncorrected $Paco_2$ was kept at 40 mm Hg (alpha-stat), cerebral metabolism (measured as cerebral oxygen consumption) decreased with cooling to 25 per cent of normothermic levels, whereas cerebral blood flow was reduced to only 58 per cent of normal. With alpha-stat acid–base regulation, cerebral blood flow correlated with cerebral oxygen consumption during hypothermia but was independent of cerebral perfusion pressure over 20 to 100 mm Hg, showing intact autoregulation. In contrast, when corrected $Paco_2$ was maintained at 40 mm Hg (pH-stat), cerebral oxygen consumption and cerebral blood flow varied independently and cerebral blood flow changed significantly with cerebral perfusion pressure. These studies have been criticized because of the methodology used to measure cerebral blood flow and await confirmation by studies using other methods. Use of [133]xenon injected into the aortic root may not yield accurate measurements of cerebral blood flow, and, if not, the derived cerebral metabolic rate values are also problematic in such studies.[40]

Subject to these possible limitations, these preliminary studies suggest that pH-stat defeats effective cerebral autoregulation during hypothermia to maintain constant and high levels of brain blood flow in the face of variations in perfusion pressure and metabolic rate. When pH-stat was used in these studies, cerebral blood flow was relatively high and probably excessive for the markedly decreased cerebral metabolic rates during hypothermia. Unnecessarily high cerebral flows may subject the microcirculation of the brain to excessive amounts of blood microaggregrates and other bypass-related factors, causing endothelial damage, and also might increase intracerebral pressure.

In addition to these probable effects of acid–base regulation on coupling of cerebral metabolism and blood flow, preservation of cerebral microcirculation and stores of brain high-energy phosphates are directly affected by pH during hypothermia. In brain, hypothermia increases pH_i and markedly inhibits development of intracellular acidosis with ischemia, preserving intracellular concentrations of adenosine triphosphate (ATP) during ischemia.[41, 42] Although not yet studied experimentally, lowering of pH_i with pH-stat regulation may inhibit this mechanism of hypothermic protection. In addition, when brain perfusate is alkalinized during normothermic anoxia, brain microcirculation is much better preserved than with normal pH.[43] In this study, hypothermia to 20° C preserved brain microcirculation to a much better degree during anoxia, but this improvement was largely lost when blood pH was acidified to levels approximating those seen with pH-stat regulation.[43]

An interesting incidental finding in a study of somatosensory evoked potentials during hypothermic circulatory arrest in children was that alpha-stat pH levels in blood at onset of circulatory arrest were associated with quickest recovery of cortical evoked potentials on rewarming, whereas *more alkaline* pH values were linearly related to prolonged evoked potential recovery time, suggesting less adequate cerebral preservation.[44] In the same study, pH during reperfusion and rewarming demonstrated no relation with return of cortical evoked potential activity. Unfortunately there are no studies of effects of different acid–base regulation on neurologic outcome after hypothermic bypass to support such incidental observations. Anecdotal reports of use of alpha-stat strategy present *impressions* of improved myocardial function and absence of cerebral complications, but these are hardly controlled, comparative studies.[45]

Heart

The heart is frequently subjected to periods of ischemia with aortic cross-clamping during hypothermia. However, when cardioplegia is used during periods of myocardial ischemia, cardioplegia solution controls extracellular pH. Acid–base regulation of cardioplegia solution then becomes the issue. The effects of acid–base regulation of blood again become important only on reperfusion.

It has been well documented in experimental animals during ischemia that acidosis (coronary sinus blood) develops in normothermic and hypothermic heart and is associated with decreased contractility on reperfusion. Alkalinization of blood before occlusion has significantly decreased such acidosis and resulted in better contractility on reperfusion.[46-48]

Extracellular pH (coronary sinus blood) falls markedly with 1 hour of ischemia, even with topical cooling of heart to 16° C.[49] In this study, pH of blood at 30° C reperfusing the heart after 1 hour of ischemia was shown to be critical for recovery of left ventricular performance, with pH of 7.7 to 7.9 (corrected) being optimal. This corresponds to moderately alkaline acid–base regulation compared with alpha-stat. Becker et al.[50] also studied myocardial effects of acid–base regulation more alkaline than alpha-stat. During surface cooling, alkaline pH (7.7 uncorrected) resulted in improved cardiac output compared with pure alpha-stat management (7.4 uncorrected). With alkaline management, recovery of myocardial performance after 1 hour of circulatory arrest and cardioplegic protection was 50 per cent better than with alpha-stat management, approximating preischemic control performance.

In nonischemic hearts, alpha-stat appears superior to pH-stat in some studies but not in others. One study showed no effect of alpha-stat versus pH-stat in perfusate blood on performance of isolated hearts, suggesting that intracellular buffering efficiency and membrane ion pumps can compensate for relatively wide ranges of extracellular pH.[51] In contrast, McConnell et al.[52] showed that use of alpha-stat blood regulation (pH 7.72, corrected) compared with pH-stat regulation (pH 7.4, corrected) in dogs cooled to 28° C resulted in significant increases in total left ventricular coronary flow, especially subendocardially, as well as increased myocardial oxygen consumption, lactate usage, and left ventricular performance curves.

Cardiac electrophysiology appears to be affected by acid–base regulation. Two studies showed that pH-stat regulation during hypothermia *decreased* the electrical stability of the heart, resulting in high incidence of spontaneous ventricular fibrillation in dogs.[53, 54] The electrical stability of the heart during hypothermia was significantly *increased* using alpha-stat blood regulation in one of these studies.[53] In a study of consecutive patients (not randomized), use of pH-stat management during cooling on bypass to 24° C resulted in a 40 per cent incidence of ventricular fibrillation before aortic cross-clamping, significantly higher than the 20 per cent incidence seen using alpha-stat management.[55]

Intracellular pH in myocardium of experimental animals decreases with both normothermic and hypothermic ischemia and increases with cooling.[56, 57] The rate of development of intracellular acidosis is markedly inhibited by hypothermia in ischemic myocardium. Ischemic skeletal muscle behaves similarly when cooled.[58] Although hypothermia itself

TABLE 1–1. DIFFERENT HYPOTHERMIC ACID–BASE REGULATORY STRATEGIES

Strategy	Aim	Total CO_2 Content	pH and $Paco_2$ Maintenance	Intracellular State	Alpha-imidazole and Buffering	Enzyme Structure and Function	Cerebral Blood Flow and Coupling	Effect on Ischemic Tissue
pH-stat	Constant pH	Increases	Normal corrected values	Acidotic (excess H^+)	Excess (+) charge Buffering decreased	Altered and activity decreased	Flow close to normothermic ? Flow and metabolism uncoupled	? Lessens hypothermic protection
Alpha-stat	Constant OH^-/H^+	Constant	Normal uncorrected values	Neutral (H^+ = OH^-)	Constant net charge Buffering constant	Normal and activity maximal	Flow decreases (appropriate) ? Flow and metabolism coupled	? Allows full hypothermic protection
Alkaline	Alkaline pH	Decreases	Alkaline and hypocapneic uncorrected values	? Alkalotic (excess OH^+)	Decreased (+) charge Buffering increased	Altered and activity decreased	? Flow decreases ? Flow and metabolism coupling	? Augments hypothermic protection

clearly inhibits development of intracellular myocardial acidosis, cardioplegia at various levels of pH had relatively little effect on development of this acidosis during hypothermia, especially at temperatures less than 20° C, even using markedly alkalotic cardioplegia.[51] This suggests that during deep hypothermia, pH of the perfusate has relatively little effect on pH_i, possibly indicating local control. In contrast, other experimental studies have shown that during hypothermia, use of a slightly acidotic cardioplegia containing glutamate produces mild intracellular acidosis and results in better preservation of ATP stores and functional recovery.[59]

In patients, progressive decreases in myocardial pH_i during aortic cross-clamping at myocardial temperatures of 10° to 15° C have been demonstrated. The pH_i is progressively decreased below pN (the starting pH_i) as ischemic time continues, suggesting the importance of alpha-stat intracellular regulation in human myocardial tissue.[60] Blood cardioplegia maintained pH_i closer to pN during ischemia than did crystalloid cardioplegia, and resulted in significantly less inotropic and mechanical support requirements in patients.[60]

No coherent pattern emerges from these cardiac studies except perhaps to suggest that acid–base regulation during hypothermia may be relatively more important in ischemic myocardial tissue. By introducing a third alternative acid–base regulatory scheme, one which is alkaline compared with alpha-stat, the question is only further complicated (Table 1–1).

CONCLUSIONS

What type of acid–base regulation should be followed during hypothermic CPB? No firm conclusion can be reached based on currently available data. Simplicity of implementation, theoretical rationale, probable maintenance of coupling between cerebral blood flow and metabolism, and perhaps better preservation of ischemic myocardium would suggest that alpha-stat regulation is probably better under most conditions. However, factors such as availability of different substrates, ionic milieu, level of tissue perfusion, and conditions of reperfusion after ischemia may well act synergistically to modify effects of acid–base regulation under various clinical circumstances. Without knowing more about linkage between intracellular and extracellular acid–base regulation in various human tissues, these possibilities cannot be evaluated. Ultimately, until well-controlled studies of both organ function and outcome using various systems of acid–base regulation during hypothermic bypass are performed in humans, the complex dilemma of proper acid–base regulation during hypothermia will not be solved. It is hoped that this review will have convinced the reader, at the least, that the subject is complex and worthy of careful thought and study.

References

1. Moore B: The cause of the exquisite sensitivity of living cells to changes in hydrogen and hydroxyl-ion concentration. J Physiol (London) 53:57–58, 1919.
2. Rosenthal TB: The effect of temperature on the pH of blood and plasma in vitro. J Biol Chem 173:25–34, 1948.
3. Severinghaus JW: Respiration and hypothermia. Ann NY Acad Sci 80:384–394, 1959.
4. Severinghaus JW: Blood gas calculator. J Appl Physiol 21:1108–1116, 1966.
5. Austin JH, Cullen GE: Hydrogen ion concentration of the blood in health and disease. Medicine 4:275–343, 1925.
6. Austin JH, Sunderman FW, Camack JG: Studies in serum electrolytes. II. The electrolyte composition and the pH of serum of a poikilothermous animal at different temperature. J Biol Chem 72:677–685, 1927.
7. Robin ED: Relationship between temperature and plasma pH and carbon dioxide tension in the turtle. Nature 195:249–250, 1962.
8. Reeves RB: Temperature-induced changes in blood acid–base status: pH and Pa_{CO_2} in a binary buffer. J Appl Physiol 40:752–761, 1976.
9. Reeves RB: Temperature-induced changes in blood acid–base status: Donnan r_{Cl} and red cell volume. J Appl Physiol 40:762–767, 1976.
10. Rahn H: Body temperature and acid–base regulation. Pneumonologie 151:87, 1974.
11. Howell BJ, Baumgardner FW, Bondi K, Rahn H: Acid–base balance in cold-blooded vertebrates as a function of body temperature. Am J Physiol 218:600–606, 1970.
12. Reeves RB: The interaction of body temperature and acid–base balance in ectothermic vertebrates. Ann Rev Physiol 39:559–586, 1977.
13. Rahn H, Reeves RB, Howell BJ: Hydrogen ion regulation, temperature and evolution. Am Rev Resp Dis 112:165–172, 1975.
14. White FN: A comparative physiological approach to hypothermia. J Thorac Cardiovasc Surg 82:821–828, 1981.
15. Swan H: The importance of acid–base management for cardiac and cerebral preservation during open heart operations. Surg Gynecol Obstet 158:391–414, 1984.
16. Ream AK, Reitz BA, Silverberg G: Temperature correction of p_{CO_2} and pH in estimating acid–base status: An example of the emperor's new clothes? Anesthesiology 56:41–44, 1982.
17. Marshall BE, Williams JJ: A fresh look at an old question. Anesthesiology 56:1–2, 1982.
18. Swan H: The hydroxyl-hydrogen ion concentration ratio during hypothermia. Surg Gynecol Obstet 155:897–912, 1982.
19. Davis BD: On the importance of being ionized. Arch Biochem Biophys 78:497–509, 1958.
20. Somero GN, White FN: Enzymatic consequences under alphastat regulation. In Rahn H, Prakash O (eds): Acid-Base Regulation and Body Temperature. Boston, Martinus Nijhoff, 1985, pp 55–80.
21. Howell BH, Rahn H: Regulation of acid–base balance in reptiles. In Gans C, Dawson WR (eds): Biology of the Reptilia, vol 5. London, Academic Press, 1976, pp 335–363.
22. Reeves RB, Rahn H: Patterns in vertebrate acid–base regulation. In Wood S, Lenfant C (eds): Evolution of Respiratory Processes: A Comparative Approach. New York, Marcel Dekker, 1979, pp 225–252.
23. Malan A, Wilson C, Reeves RB: Intracellular pH in cold-blooded vertebrates as a function of body temperature. Respir Physiol 28:29–47, 1976.
24. Reeves RB: What are normal acid–base conditions in man when body temperature changes? In Rahn H, Prakash O (eds): Acid–Base Regulation and Body Temperature. Boston, Martinus Nijhoff, 1985, pp 13–32.
25. White FN, Somero GN: Acid–base regulation and phospholipid adaptations to temperature: Time courses and physiological significance of modifying the milieu for protein function. Physiol Rev 62:40–90, 1982.
26. Blayo MC, Lecompte Y, Pocidalo JJ: Control of acid–base status during hypothermia in man. Respir Physiol 42:287–298, 1980.
27. Malan A: Acid–base regulation during hibernation. In Rahn H, Prakash O (eds): Acid–Base Regulation and Body Temperature. Boston, Martinus Nijhoff, 1985, pp 33–53.

28. Nuccitelli R, Heiple JM: Summary of the evidence and discussion concerning the involvement of pH_i in the control of cellular functions. In Nuccitelli R, Deamer DW (eds): Intracellular pH: Its Measurement, Regulation, and Utilization in Cellular Functions. New York, Allen R. Liss, 1982, pp 567–586.
29. Williamson JR, Safer B, Rich T, et al: Effects of acidosis on myocardial contractility and metabolism. Acta Med Scand [Suppl] 587:95–111, 1975.
30. Bickler PE: Intracellular pH in the lizard Dipsosaurus dorsalis in relation to changing body temperatures. J Physiol (London) 53:1466–1472, 1982.
31. Heisler N: Comparative aspects of acid–base regulation. In Heisler N (ed): Acid–Base Regulation in Animals. Amsterdam, Elsevier Biomedical Press, 1986, pp 397–450.
32. Boutilier RG, Glass ML, Heisler N: Blood gases, and extracellular/intracellular acid–base status as a function of temperature in the anuran amphibians xenopus laevis and bufo marinus. J Exp Biol 130:13–25, 1987.
33. Heisler N, Neumann P: The role of physico-chemical buffering and of bicarbonate transfer processes in intracellular pH regulation in response to changes of temperature in the larger spotted dogfish (Scyliorhinus stellaris). J Exp Biol 85:99–110, 1980.
34. Fox LS, Blackstone EH, Kirklin JW, et al: Relationship of brain blood flow and oxygen consumption to perfusion flow rate during profoundly hypothermic cardiopulmonary bypass. J Thorac Cardiovasc Surg 87:658–664, 1984.
35. Govier AV, Reves JG, McKay RD, et al: Factors and their influence on regional cerebral blood flow during nonpulsatile cardiopulmonary bypass. Ann Thorac Surg 38:592–600, 1984.
36. Lundar T, Lindegaard K-F, Froysaker T, et al: Cerebral carbon dioxide reactivity during nonpulsatile cardiopulmonary bypass. Ann Thorac Surg 41:525–530, 1986.
37. Prough DS, Stump DA, Roy RC, et al: Response of cerebral blood flow to changes in carbon dioxide during hypothermic cardiopulmonary bypass. Anesthesiology 64:576–581, 1986.
38. Fox LS, Blackstone EH, Kirklin JW, et al: Relationship of whole body oxygen consumption to perfusion flow rate during hypothermic cardiopulmonary bypass. J Thorac Cardiovasc Surg 83:239–248, 1982.
39. Murkin JM, Farrar JK, Tweed WA, et al: Cerebral autoregulation and flow/metabolism coupling during cardiopulmonary bypass: The influence of P_{CO_2}. Anesth Analg 66:825–830, 1987.
40. Michenfelder JD: Personal communication, 1988.
41. Norwood WI, Norwood CR, Ingwall JS, et al: Hypothermic circulatory arrest: 31-phosphorus nuclear magnetic resonance of isolated perfused neonatal rat brain. J Thorac Cardiovasc Surg 78:823–830, 1979.
42. Norwood WI, Norwood CR: Influence of hypothermia on intracellular pH during anoxia. Am J Physiol 243:C62–C65, 1982.
43. Norwood WI, Norwood CR, Castaneda AR: Cerebral anoxia: Effect of deep hypothermia and pH. Surgery 86:203–209, 1979.
44. Coles JG, Taylor MJ, Pearce JM, et al: Cerebral monitoring of somatosensory evoked potential during profoundly hypothermic circulatory arrest. Circulation 70(suppl I):I96-I102, 1984.
45. Matthews AJ, Stead AL, Abbott TR: Acid–base control during hypothermia. Anaesthesia 39:649–654, 1984.
46. Austen EG: Experimental studies on the effects of acidosis and alkalosis on myocardial function after aortic occlusion. J Surg Res 5:191–194, 1965.
47. Wang H, Katz RL: Effects of changes in coronary blood pH on the heart. Circ Res 17:114–122, 1965.
48. Ebert PA, Greenfield LJ, Austen WG, et al: The relationship of blood pH during profound hypothermia to subsequent myocardial infarction. Surg Gynecol Obstet 114:357–362, 1962.
49. Follette DM, Fey K, Livesay J, et al: Studies on myocardial reperfusion injury-I. Surgery 82:149–155, 1977.
50. Becker H, Vinten–Johansen J, Buckberg GD, et al: Myocardial damage caused by keeping pH 7.40 during systemic deep hypothermia. J Thorac Cardiovasc Surg 82:810–820, 1981.

51. Sinet M, Muffat–Joly M, Bendaace T, et al: Maintaining blood at 7.4 during hypothermia has no significant effect on work of the isolated rat heart. Anesthesiology 62:582–587, 1985.
52. McConnell DH, White FN, Nelson RL, et al: Importance of alkalosis in maintenance of "ideal" blood pH during hypothermia. Surg Forum 26:263–265, 1975.
53. Swain JA, White FN, Peters RM: The effect of pH on the hypothermic ventricular fibrillation threshold. J Thorac Cardiovasc Surg 87:445–451, 1984.
54. Gillen JP, Vogel MFX, Holterman RK, et al: Ventricular fibrillation during orotracheal intubation of hypothermic dogs. Ann Emerg Med 15:412–416, 1986.
55. Kroncke GM, Nichols RD, Mendenhall JT, et al: Ectothermic philosophy of acid–base balance to prevent fibrillation during hypothermia. Arch Surg 121:303–304, 1986.
56. Lange R, Cavanough AC, Zierler M, et al: The relative importance of alkalinity, temperature, and the washout effect of bicarbonate-buffered, multidose cardioplegic solution. Circulation 70 (suppl I) : I75–I83, 1984.
57. Wilson GJ, Robertson JM, Walters FJM, et al: Intramyocardial pH during elective arrest of the heart: Relative effects of hypothermia versus potassium cardioplegia on anaerobic metabolism. Ann Thorac Surg 30:472–481, 1980.
58. Osterman AL, Heppenstall RB, Sapega AA: Muscle ischemia and hypothermia: A bioenergetic study using phosphorous nuclear magnetic resonance spectroscopy. J Trauma 24:811–817, 1984.
59. Bernard M, Menasche P, Canioni P, et al: Influence of the pH of cardioplegic solutions on intracellular pH, high energy phosphates, and postarrest performance. J Thorac Cardiovasc Surg 90:235–242, 1985.
60. Khuri SF, Warner KG, Josa M, et al: The superiority of continuous cold blood cardioplegia in the metabolic protection of the hypertrophied human heart. J Thorac Cardiovasc Surg 95:442–454, 1988.

CHAPTER 2

THE INFLUENCE OF CARDIOPULMONARY BYPASS ON CEREBRAL PHYSIOLOGY AND FUNCTION

IAN R. THOMSON

Properly conducted cardiopulmonary bypass (CPB) maintains cerebral function and viability by ensuring adequate regional delivery of oxygen and substrate, and removal of CO_2 and metabolic waste products. Recent studies indicate that the manner in which perfusion is conducted significantly influences cerebral blood flow (CBF) and metabolism. This new information is relevant to controversies regarding the optimum acid–base management strategy, mean arterial pressure (MAP), perfusion flow rate (Q), and perfusion pattern (pulsatile or nonpulsatile) that are appropriate for maintenance of brain viability during CPB. Unequivocal resolution of these controversies awaits prospective clinical trials examining the influence of perfusion-related variables on neurologic outcome. This discussion will (a) examine the influence of perfusion on CBF and metabolism, (b) assess the relation between the conduct of perfusion and neurologic outcome, and (c) make recommendations regarding the appropriate conduct of bypass.

CEREBRAL BLOOD FLOW AND METABOLISM

Normal Cerebral Physiology

In awake humans CBF is 45 to 50 ml • 100 g^{-1} • min^{-1}, and cerebral oxygen consumption ($CMRO_2$) 3.0 ml • 100 g^{-1} • min^{-1}.[1] Normally the major determinant of CBF is $CMRO_2$. This linkage is called "flow-metabolism coupling." Cerebrovascular "autoregulation" is one manifestation of flow-metabolism coupling. Autoregulation describes the phenomenon whereby CBF is normally independent of cerebral perfusion pressure (CPP) over the range of 50 to 150 mm Hg. CPP is the hydrostatic pressure gradient that promotes CBF, and is calculated as the difference between MAP and intracranial pressure (ICP) (CPP = MAP − ICP). At CPP's outside the autoregulatory range, CBF is pressure-dependent (i.e., directly related to CPP). When CPP decreases below the lower autoregulatory threshold of 50 mm Hg, CBF decreases progressively. ICP is seldom measured during bypass. Therefore, clinicians and investigators often use MAP interchangeably with CPP. This practice involves tenuous and often invalid assumptions about the magnitude of ICP and the absence of significant cerebrovascular occlusive disease.[2, 3]

Flow-metabolism coupling explains the effects of most intravenous anesthetics, temperature (T), and arterial oxygen content (C_aO_2) on CBF. For example, intravenous anesthetics[1] (except ketamine) and hypothermia[4] decrease both $CMRO_2$ and CBF. Decreases in C_aO_2 caused by hypoxemia[5] or hemodilution[6] increase CBF. CO_2 affects CBF independently of $CMRO_2$. CBF increases approximately 2 ml • 100 g^{-1} • min^{-1} for each 1 mm Hg increment in Pa_{CO_2}.[7] Unphysiologically high Pa_{CO_2} levels block autoregulation and produce a "pressure-dependent" cerebral circulation.

Perfusion-related Influences on CBF and $CMRO_2$

The response of $CMRO_2$ and CBF to CPB is variable, and depends on the manner in which perfusion is conducted. Widely differing perfusion protocols used in different institutions were developed in the absence of reliable data pertaining to their cerebral effects. Recently, however, several groups of investigators have measured CBF and/or $CMRO_2$ before, during, and after CPB in humans undergoing cardiac surgery.[2, 3, 8–17] These studies define the influence of anesthesia, temperature, acid–base management, Q, MAP, and pulsation on cerebral physiology. Each of these variables is considered below.

Anesthetic Effects

Volatile anesthetics, opioids, and sedative-hypnotics are commonly administered to patients before and during bypass. These agents depress cerebral function and cause dose-related reductions in $CMRO_2$.[1] In general, intravenous anesthetics do not alter flow-metabolism coupling, and their administration reduces both $CMRO_2$ and CBF. For example, Murkin et al.[14] (Figs. 2–1 and 2–2) measured $CMRO_2$ and CBF before bypass in patients undergoing coronary artery surgery (CAS) under fentanyl (100 μg • kg) and diazepam (0.5 mg/kg) anesthesia. Cerebral oxygen consumption was 1.67 ml • 100 g^{-1} • min^{-1}, and CBF was 25 ml • 100 g^{-1} • min^{-1} (i.e., about 50 per cent of anticipated awake values). However, volatile

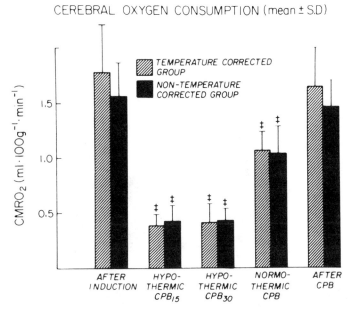

CEREBRAL OXYGEN CONSUMPTION (mean ± S.D.)

Figure 2–1. Effect of acid–base management on cerebral oxygen consumption in patients undergoing coronary artery surgery under high-dose fentanyl–diazepam anesthesia and hypothermic nonpulsatile cardiopulmonary bypass. Acid–base management did not influence oxygen consumption. Effects of anesthesia, hypothermia, and nonpulsatile flow are discussed in the text. ‡ indicates $p < .001$ versus control. (From Murkin JM, Farrar JK, Tweed A, et al: Cerebral autoregulation and flow/metabolism coupling during cardiopulmonary bypass: The influence of $Paco_2$. Anesth Analg 66:825, 1987, with permission.)

anesthetics uncouple flow and metabolism, and cause cerebral hyperperfusion relative to $CMRO_2$. Murkin et al. found that isoflurane anesthesia reduced $CMRO_2$ to the same extent as fentanyl–diazepam but did not reduce CBF.[15]

Hypothermia

Systemic hypothermia is usually used during CPB. Hypothermia reduces $CMRO_2$ and, theoretically, may protect the brain. The effect of hypothermic bypasss on $CMRO_2$ is superimposed on that of prebypass anesthesia, and the combination reduces $CMRO_2$ profoundly. During high-dose fentanyl–diazepam anesthesia, Murkin et al.[14] (Fig. 2–1) found that $CMRO_2$ was 0.42 ml • 100 g^{-1} • min^{-1} during hypothermic (26.6° C) nonpulsatile CPB. During normothermic (36.9° C) bypass, $CMRO_2$ was 1.05 ml • 100 g^{-1} • min^{-1}. Thus each 10° C change in temperature altered $CMRO_2$ by a factor (Q_{10}) of 2.5. This value for cerebral Q_{10} is comparable to that obtained for the whole body by other investigators.[18, 19] During hypothermic (26.6° C) bypass and fentanyl (100 μg • kg^{-1}) anesthesia, induction of electroencephalographic burst-suppression with either thio-

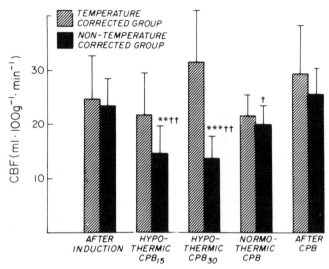

Figure 2–2. Effect of acid–base management on cerebral blood flow in patients undergoing coronary artery surgery under high-dose fentanyl–diazepam anesthesia and hypothermic nonpulsatile cardiopulmonary bypass. In the temperature corrected group, CO_2 was added during hypothermia to obtain a "normal" temperature-corrected $Paco_2$ of 40 mm Hg (pH-stat management). In the non-temperature corrected group, CO_2 was not added, and uncorrected $Paco_2$ was 40 mm Hg (alpha-stat management). pH-stat management caused cerebral hyperperfusion during hypothermic bypass.* indicates p <.005 between groups. (From Murkin JM, Farrar JK, Tweed A, et al: Cerebral autoregulation and flow/metabolism coupling during cardiopulmonary bypass: The influence of $Paco_2$. Anesth Analg 66:825, 1987, with permission.)

pental or isoflurane reduced $CMRO_2$ below 0.3 ml $\cdot$ 100 g $\cdot$ min^{-1}, compared with 0.41 ml $\cdot$ 100 g^{-1} $\cdot$ min^{-1} in control patients (p <.05).[16] Although changes in $CMRO_2$ during hypothermic CPB are predictable, the CBF response is critically dependent on the acid–base management strategy used.

Carbon Dioxide (See also Chapter 1)

When blood is drawn from a hypothermic patient, arterial pH (pH$_a$) and $Paco_2$ are measured at 37° C and must be mathematically corrected to obtain in vivo pH$_a$ and $Paco_2$.[20] Because CO_2 is more soluble at low temperature, $Paco_2$ falls and pH$_a$ rises in vivo during hypothermia if blood CO_2 content remains constant. To prevent this apparent "hypocapnia" and "alkalosis," some clinicians add CO_2 to the gas entering the oxygenator. If sufficient CO_2 is added, temperature-corrected pH$_a$ and $Paco_2$ values during hypothermic bypass will be similar to the usual normothermic values. This "pH-stat" (i.e., constant pH$_a$) acid–base strategy assumes that typical normothermic pH_a and $Paco_2$ values are also appropriate during hypothermia. An alternative "alpha-stat" acid–base strategy has been advocated.[21] This approach duplicates the acid–base physiology of poikilothermic animals during hypothermic bypass in humans. Poikilotherms maintain relatively constant blood CO_2 content over a wide temperature range.[22, 23] Therefore, during hypothermia their in vivo $Paco_2$ decreases while pH_a increases. This response maintains a constant ratio of hydrogen to hydroxyl ions in blood, and may be important for optimal function of cellular proteins. Maintenance of constant blood CO_2 content during hypothermia implies that when pH_a and $Paco_2$ are measured at 37° C, "normal" uncorrected values will be found.[21]

Both of these acid–base management strategies are currently used during hypothermic CPB in humans. Murkin et al. (Fig. 2–2) demonstrated that the CBF response to hypothermia is profoundly influenced by acid–base management.[14] They studied patients undergoing CAS under hypothermic, nonpulsatile CPB. In one group (pH-stat), CO_2 was added to the gases entering the oxygenator, so that temperature-corrected $Paco_2$ approximated 40 mm Hg at 26° C. In the other group (alpha-stat), management was similar, except that CO_2 was not added during hypothermia, and temperature-corrected $Paco_2$ was 26 mm Hg (uncorrected $Paco_2$ approximated 40 mm Hg). Cerebral oxygen consumption was markedly reduced in both groups at low temperature. Adding CO_2 (pH-stat) during hypothermia increased CBF dramatically compared with normothermic values, causing cerebral hyperperfusion relative to oxygen demand. In contrast, when CO_2 was not added during hypothermia (alpha-stat), CBF fell appropriately, given the decreased $CMRO_2$ and extent of hemodilution. With pH-stat management, CBF was independent of $CMRO_2$ and C_aO_2, but correlated with MAP (Fig. 2–3). Thus adding CO_2 during hypothermia abolishes flow-metabolism coupling and autoregulation, and creates a pressure-dependent cerebral circulation. Conversely, with alpha-stat management, CBF correlated with $CMRO_2$ and C_aO_2 but was independent of MAP, implying preservation of flow-metabolism coupling, and autoregulation.

Murkin's work resolves a controversy regarding the overall CBF response to hypothermic CPB. Using pH-stat management, Henriksen et al.[8] and Lundar et al.[2, 3] reported cerebral hyperperfusion, and a pressure-dependent cerebral circulation during hypothermic CPB. Conversely, Govier et al.[11] and Prough et al.[12] found that CBF was reduced and autoregulation preserved when alpha-stat management was used. Henriksen originally explained the cerebral hyperperfusion he observed during CPB as a pathophysiologic response to diffuse cerebrovascular microembolism.[8] However, this "luxury-perfusion" is likely entirely attributable to pH-stat acid–base management.[10, 12, 14]

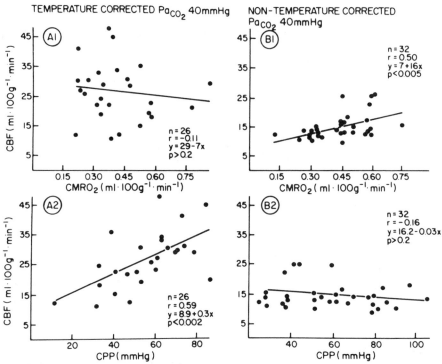

Figure 2–3. Influence of acid–base management on the correlations between cerebral blood flow and both cerebral perfusion pressure and cerebral oxygen consumption. In the temperature corrected group (A1 and A2), CO_2 was added during hypothermia to obtain a "normal" temperature-corrected Pa_{CO_2} of 40 mm Hg (pH-stat management). In the non-temperature corrected group (B1 and B2), CO_2 was not added, and uncorrected Pa_{CO_2} was 40 mm Hg (alpha-stat management). pH-stat management appears to abolish flow-metabolism coupling and autoregulation, whereas alpha-stat management preserved them. With alpha-stat management, the lower autoregulatory threshold appears to be extended to nearly 20 mm Hg. (From Murkin JM, Farrar JK, Tweed A, et al: Cerebral autoregulation and flow/metabolism coupling during cardiopulmonary bypass: The influence of Pa_{CO_2}. Anesth Analg 66:825, 1987, with permission.)

Measurement of CBF during hypothermic bypass may be a "litmus test" for comparing acid–base management strategies. By this criterion, alpha-stat management appears to be the more physiologic approach. However, the influence of acid–base management on cerebral function after bypass has not been prospectively investigated. Theoretically, cerebral hyperperfusion associated with pH-stat management might be hazardous. Potential consequences of hyperperfusion include disruption of the cerebral microcirculation, increased ICP, production of a cerebrovascular "steal" in patients with cerebrovascular disease, and preferential delivery of microemboli to the brain. Despite a lack of outcome data, the weight of evidence currently militates against the addition of CO_2 to gases entering the oxygenator during hypothermic bypass.

Cerebral Perfusion Pressure

Alpha-stat acid–base management appears to preserve cerebral flow-metabolism coupling and autoregulation during hypothermic CPB in humans. However, a controversy has arisen regarding the extent of the autoregulatory range. Does the cerebral circulation become pressure-dependent when CPP falls below 50 mm Hg, or is the CPP threshold extended to lower values during hypothermia? In the absence of ICP measurements, what is the critical MAP value below which autoregulation fails? These questions are important because some institutions conduct "low-flow low-pressure" bypass in which MAP is deliberately kept at or below the normothermic autoregulatory threshold of 50 mm Hg.[24]

Using [133]xenon washout, Govier et al.[11] performed the first CBF measurements in humans during hypothermic CPB, using alpha-stat acid–base management. Regression analysis of pooled data from 69 patients undergoing CAS indicated that CBF correlated with nasopharyngeal T and $PaCO_2$ but was independent of MAP. Therefore, they concluded that flow-metabolism coupling and autoregulation were intact. Because individual MAP values ranged from 30 to 110 mm Hg, Govier et al. further concluded that "during hypothermic CPB the lower limit of autoregulation appears to be as low as 30 mm Hg," and that "pharmacologic support is not necessary to maintain a constant CBF between a MAP of 30 and 110 mm Hg." Based on actual $CMRO_2$ measurements and a similar regression analysis (Fig. 2–3), Murkin et al.[14] similarly concluded that "autoregulation appears to be intact over a range of cerebral perfusion pressures from 20 to 100 mm Hg." Although tenable, these conclusions remain unproved, since neither experiment prospectively tested the hypothesis that the autoregulatory threshold is altered during hypothermic bypass, or assessed outcome as a function of perfusion pressure. Because most CBF determinations were at MAP or CPP values within the usual autoregulatory range of 50 to 100 mm Hg, a correlation would not be expected, even if CBF were pressure-dependent below 50 mm Hg. To prove a shift in the autoregulatory threshold with hypothermia, CPP must be varied over a wide range in individual patients, during both normo- and hypothermia.

Theoretically, a shift in autoregulatory threshold might be anticipated during hypothermia (Fig. 2–4). Presumably, the autoregulatory plateau in the relation between CBF and CPP is determined by $CMRO_2$ and C_aO_2. The level of this plateau is directly proportional to $CMRO_2$ and inversely proportional to C_aO_2. The autoregulatory plateau would be expected to decline during hypothermia, despite moderate hemodilution, because of

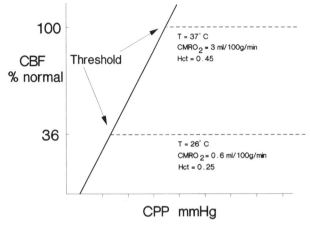

Figure 2–4. Theoretical effect of fentanyl–diazepam anesthesia and hypothermic bypass on the autoregulatory threshold. The solid line represents the pressure-flow relation of the maximally vasodilated cerebral circulation. The autoregulatory threshold is the point where the autoregulatory plateau (dashed lines) intersects the maximally vasodilated curve. The height of the plateau is directly proportional to $CMRO_2$ and inversely proportional to C_aO_2. Hypothermic bypass shifts the autoregulatory threshold leftward to a lower value.

the marked reduction in $CMRO_2$. The lower autoregulatory threshold can be perceived as the point at which the plateau intersects the pressure-dependent, maximally dilated pressure-flow curve. Lowering $CMRO_2$, and thus the autoregulatory plateau, shifts the point of intersection, and the autoregulatory threshold, to a lower pressure.

On the other hand, some data suggest that the lower autoregulatory threshold is not substantially altered by hypothermic bypass. Fox et al.[19] measured jugular venous O_2 saturation $(S_{jv}O_2)$ in ten cardiac surgical patients undergoing hypothermic (T = 20° C) CPB, with alpha-stat pH management. In each patient $S_{jv}O_2$ was measured at four systemic blood flows, instituted at random, between 0.25 and 2.0 $l \cdot min^{-1} \cdot m^{-2}$. MAP fell from 52 to 8 mm Hg as Q was decreased from 2.0 to 0.25 $l \cdot min^{-1} \cdot m^{-2}$. Jugular venous O_2 saturation fell progressively from 82 to 25 per cent as Q and MAP were reduced (Fig. 2–5). Although CBF was not measured, the data suggest that MAP values of less than 50 mm Hg are below the autoregulatory threshold. When MAP fell below 50 mm Hg, CBF apparently decreased, necessitating increased O_2 extraction from arterial blood. This was manifested as a decrease in $S_{jv}O_2$.

Feddersen et al.[13] provide further evidence of an unchanged autoregulatory threshold during hypothermic CPB. They studied patients, without evident cerebrovascular disease, undergoing CAS under hypothermic (T = 28° C) bypass, and alpha-stat acid–base management. Fentanyl, 15 to 20 μg/kg, and droperidol, 100 μg/kg, were given before bypass. Patients received either prostacyclin, 50 $ng \cdot kg^{-1} \cdot min^{-1}$, or placebo during CPB.

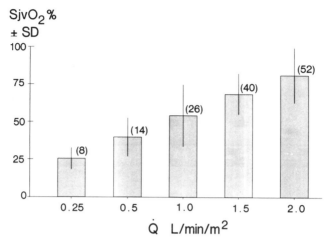

Figure 2–5. Effect of perfusion flow rate (Q) on jugular venous oxygen saturation ($S_{jv}O_2$) in humans undergoing hypothermic (20° C) nonpulsatile cardiopulmonary bypass with alpha-stat pH management. Figures in parentheses indicate mean arterial pressure (mm Hg) corresponding to the specific flow rate. The data indicate a pressure-passive cerebral circulation at arterial pressures below 50 mm Hg. (Drawn from data in Fox LS, Blackstone EH, Kirklin JW, et al: Relationship of whole body oxygen consumption to perfusion flow rate during hypothermic cardiopulmonary bypass. J Thorac Cardiovasc Surg 83:239, 1982.)

During the first hour of bypass (Fig. 2–6), MAP averaged 30 mm Hg in the prostacyclin group and 60 to 80 mm Hg in the placebo group. CBF was significantly lower (24 versus 34 ml • 100 g^{-1} • min^{-1}) in patients given prostacyclin, presumably because of the hypotension. This indicates that the MAP of 30 mm Hg in the prostacyclin group was substantially below the autoregulatory threshold. Sodium nitroprusside (SNP) was used to control hypertension and may have increased CBF in the placebo group as bypass progressed. However, the use of SNP does not explain the intergroup difference in CBF seen after 10 minutes of hypothermic bypass, when MAP was 60 mm Hg in the placebo group. The relative cerebral hypoperfusion in the prostacyclin group did not impair oxygen delivery, since $CMRO_2$ during hypothermic bypass was identical (1.0 ml • 100 g^{-1} • min^{-1}) in both prostacyclin and placebo groups. The prostacyclin patients compensated for lower CBF with increased O_2 extraction. Somatosensory evoked potentials (SEPS) were also unaltered by prostacyclin-induced hypotension, despite a widened C_aO_2 difference.[25] Feddersen's patients were not as cold or as deeply anaesthetized as those of Murkin et al., and thus their $CMRO_2$ was higher (1.0 versus 0.42 ml • 100 g^{-1} • min^{-1}). This may explain the apparent difference in autoregulatory threshold between the two studies.

Perfusion Flow Rate

Little information is available regarding the influence of Q on CBF and metabolism during hypothermic bypass in humans. Fox et al.[19] found

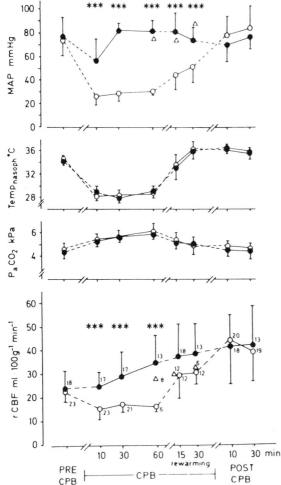

Figure 2–6. Comparison of mean arterial pressure (MAP), arterial carbon dioxide tension ($PaCO_2$) (not temperature-corrected), temperature, and cerebral blood flow (CBF) in patients given prostacyclin (open circles) and controls (closed circles). Open triangles correspond to patients in whom prostacyclin was stopped after 30 minutes on bypass. Prostacyclin reduced MAP during bypass to 30 mm Hg. This was associated with a significant reduction in CBF compared with controls, indicating that 30 mm Hg MAP is below the threshold of autoregulation. *** indicates p <.001 between groups. (From Feddersen K, Arén C, Nilsson NJ, Rådegran K: Cerebral blood flow and metabolism during cardiopulmonary bypass with special reference to effects of hypertension induced by prostacyclin. Ann Thorac Surg 41:395–400, 1986, with permission.)

that Q was the major determinant of arterial pressure, and below 1.8 l • min^{-1} • m^{-2} correlated well with $S_{jv}O_2$ (r = .72, p <.0001). Without pharmacologic support, MAP often fell below 30 mm Hg when Q was less than 1.2 l • min^{-1} • m^{-2}. Govier et al.[11] noted a borderline significant (p = .06) positive correlation between CBF and Q after stepwise regression analysis of pooled data from 67 patients. In ten patients Govier et al. varied Q between 1.3 and 2.0 l • min^{-1} • m^{-2}, and found no correlation between CBF and Q. However, MAP was kept above 45 mm Hg in this subgroup.

Rebeyka et al.[26] measured SEPS and cortical adenosine triphosphate (ATP) concentrations during hypothermic nonpulsatile CPB in dogs, as

Q was decreased from 2.0 to 0.25 l • min^{-1} • m^{-2}. Cortical ATP concentrations decreased significantly as Q declined. The SEPS were unchanged when Q was 1.0 l • min^{-1} • m^{-2} (MAP = 40 mm Hg). Increased latency of SEPS was apparent at Q = 0.5 l • min^{-1} • m^{-2} (MAP = 22 mm Hg), and SEPS were absent in all but one dog when Q was reduced to 0.25 l • min^{-1} • m^{-2}. In dogs undergoing nonpulsatile CPB at 20° C, Miyamoto et al.[27] found that $CMRO_2$ was maintained until Q was reduced below 30 ml • kg^{-1}. These data suggest that during bypass at 20° C, and without pharmacologic support of MAP, a minimum Q of 1 to 1.2 l • min^{-1} • m^{-2} is required to maintain cerebral oxygen delivery.

Pulsatile Versus Nonpulsatile Perfusion

Although flow-metabolism coupling is apparently intact during hypothermic CPB when alpha-stat acid–base management and intravenous anesthesia are used, there is indirect evidence that nonpulsatile perfusion may not meet cerebral oxygen requirements. Murkin et al.[14] (see Fig. 2–1) noted that after rewarming, $CMRO_2$ was decreased 30 per cent during normothermic nonpulsatile perfusion compared with similar measurements before or after bypass. In another study the same authors noted an immediate 37 per cent decrease in $CMRO_2$ (compared with prebypass controls) on institution of normothermic nonpulsatile bypass in patients undergoing arrhythmia surgery.[17] However, neither study directly compared $CMRO_2$ during pulsatile and nonpulsatile bypass.

Animal data support the suggestion of suboptimal oxygen delivery during nonpulsatile bypass. After 2 hours of normothermic nonpulsatile bypass in pigs, Sørensen et al.[28] found that the cerebral metabolic rate for glucose (CMR_{glc}) was 47 per cent and cerebral capillary diffusing capacity 80 per cent less than similar measurements in control animals who did not undergo bypass. These data imply occlusion of the cerebral microcirculation during nonpulsatile bypass. Possible explanations include microembolism and/or critical closure of circulatory beds in the absence of pulsation. Unfortunately this experiment did not include a group of animals who underwent pulsatile bypass, so the contribution of nonpulsatile bypass flow to the decreases in $CMRO_2$ and diffusing capacity is unclear. The instantaneous decline in $CMRO_2$ observed by Murkin et al.[17] in humans perfused from membrane oxygenators suggests nonpulsation rather than microembolism as the problem. Tranmer et al.[29] actually compared pulsatile and nonpulsatile bypass in dogs with acute focal cerebral ischemia. Compared with nonpulsatile perfusion, pulsatile flow increased CBF by 19 per cent and 55 per cent, respectively, in normal and ischemic brain regions. These various data support the long-held belief that nonpulsatile flow is "unphysiologic" and may impair cerebral circulation. Prospective clinical trials are needed to clarify the influence of pulsatile flow on CMRO$_2$, CBF, and post-bypass cerebral function in humans.

CEREBRAL DAMAGE AFTER BYPASS

Manifestations and Incidence

Brain damage after CPB may present as a focal neurologic deficit, decreased level of consciousness, or a "psychiatric" disorder such as paranoia, hallucination, or delirium. Recent prospective studies (Table 2–1) indicate a disturbingly high incidence of acute cerebral dysfunction after bypass.[30-37] Because variables such as Q, MAP, acid–base management, and pulsation clearly influence CBF and CMRO$_2$, it is reasonable to hypothesize that the conduct of bypass might influence neurologic outcome. However, there are no outcome data documenting a relation between these variables and the incidence or severity of brain damage after bypass. There are two reasonable explanations for this lack of correlation. First, a significant proportion of cerebral dysfunction after bypass is unrelated to the conduct of perfusion, but rather caused by macroemboli from the operative field or by perioperative hemodynamic instability. Second, prospective clinical trials have not examined the influence of perfusion-related variables on outcome.

Factors Associated with Neurologic Dysfunction

Most reports of brain damage after CPB have first determined the incidence of complications and then attempted retrospectively to correlate neurologic outcome with clinical variables. Conclusions based on such retrospective analyses are tenuous and should be regarded circumspectly. However, the accumulated data from multiple retrospective studies may provide insight into the causes of cerebral dysfunction after bypass. Table 2–2 documents the frequency with which clinical variables

TABLE 2–1. INCIDENCE OF NEUROLOGIC DYSFUNCTION AFTER CARDIAC SURGERY

Author	Date	Surgery	Incidence (%)*
Sotaniemi	1981	OH	27
Sotaniemi	1983	OH	37
Slogoff	1982	CAS and OH	16
Breuer	1983	CAS	17
Heikkinen	1985	CAS and OH	7
Smith	1986	CAS	4
Nussmeier	1986	OH	8

OH, open-ventricle procedures; CAS, coronary artery surgery.
*Postoperative day 4–10.

TABLE 2–2. CLINICAL CORRELATES OF CEREBRAL DAMAGE AFTER CPB

Variable	Number of Citations
Duration of bypass	15
Age	9
Open-ventricle procedure	6
Preoperative neurologic deficit	5
Perioperative hypotension or low cardiac output state	5
Hypotension during bypass	3
Aortic valve surgery	2
Valvular calcification	2
Female sex	2

Reprinted with permission from Thomson IR: Problems in Anesthesia, 1:394. Philadelphia, JB Lippincott, 1987.

have been retrospectively associated with brain damage. The most frequent correlates of central nervous system dysfunction are the duration of CPB,[31, 36–49] advanced age,[32, 34, 37, 38, 42, 45–48] open-ventricle procedures,[32, 34, 39, 42, 44, 50] preexisting neurologic deficit,[34, 39, 45–47] and perioperative hypotension or low cardiac output state.[33, 38, 43, 44, 49] Retrospective studies have infrequently documented a relation between MAP during bypass and postoperative brain damage.[24, 45, 48]

Causes of Cerebral Damage

Based on the retrospective analyses discussed above, several causative mechanisms have been proposed to explain brain damage after CPB. These include global hypoperfusion, microembolism and macroembolism.

Global Cerebral Hypoperfusion

The duration of CPB is the variable most consistently associated with postoperative neurologic dysfunction. This suggests that bypass is "unphysiologic" and causes a cumulative insult to cerebral integrity as it continues. The nature of the insult is unclear, but global cerebral hypoperfusion caused by inadequate perfusion pressure and/or nonpulsatile perfusion might contribute. The increased incidence of cerebrovascular disease in the elderly might predispose them to cerebral hypoperfusion during bypass. If so, this might explain the frequent association of advanced age with cerebral dysfunction after bypass.

Generalized cerebral hypoperfusion causes a specific neurologic lesion. Infarction occurs in the vulnerable parieto-occipital "boundary-zone" where the terminal distributions of the anterior, middle, and posterior cerebral arteries meet.[51, 52] Case reports of cortical blindness,[53] upper-extremity paralysis,[54] and other deficits, accompanied by radiologic evidence of unilateral or bilateral "boundary-zone" infarction,[55] indicate that global hypoperfusion does indeed explain some cases of brain damage, especially after CAS. Unilateral boundary-zone infarction is easily confused clinically with embolic "stroke."[54]

The role of perfusion pressure during bypass in the pathogenesis of postoperative cerebral damage has been hotly debated. Retrospective analyses from recent studies indicate no association between brain damage and the duration or extent of arterial hypotension during bypass.[32, 33, 37, 42] However, this finding does not rule out low CPP during bypass as a cause of brain damage. For example, if "low-flow low-pressure" bypass were conducted routinely,[24, 42] cerebral hypoperfusion might only be apparent in the elderly or after long perfusions, and no association with MAP would be apparent. In addition, studies reporting no association between MAP and cerebral dysfunction often excluded patients with suspected cerebrovascular disease who would be "at risk" for hypoperfusion.[13, 25, 32, 37] A large prospective study is needed to determine the influence of bypass perfusion pressure on postoperative cerebral dysfunction.

Global cerebral hypoperfusion and associated cerebral dysfunction are not necessarily related to conduct of perfusion. Perioperative hypotension and/or low cardiac output state, before or after CPB, is a frequent correlate of postoperative cerebral dysfunction, especially after CAS. Breuer et al.[33] found that perioperative use of "pressors" or balloon counterpulsation was the only correlate of diffuse cerebral dysfunction after CAS. Similarly, Gardner et al.[38] noted an 8.4-fold increase in stroke after CAS when perioperative hypotension occurred.

Microembolism

Diffuse microembolism may contribute to cerebral dysfunction after CPB, and also might account for the association of damage with duration of bypass. Microbubbles produced by bubble oxygenators are not completely removed by defoaming, settling, or microfiltration.[56–58] Abnormal blood–gas and blood–plastic interfaces cause denaturation of blood proteins.[59] Lipoprotein denaturation may result in fat embolism.[60] Platelet activation causes aggregation and microvascular occlusion.[60, 61] Complement activation leads to leukocyte aggregation and microvascular sequestration.[62] Because the lungs are bypassed, microemboli enter the systemic circulation, and thus the brain, directly. Membrane oxygenators cause less platelet[63, 64] and complement[65] activation and produce fewer cerebral arterial microbubbles[66] than do bubble oxygenators. Routine use of membrane oxygenators and arterial inflow microfilters[67] might reduce microembolism and diminish cerebral dysfunction, and their influence merits further study.

Macroembolism

According to the macroembolic theory, CPB per se, does not cause the majority of postoperative cerebral damage seen in cardiac surgical patients. Rather, cerebral damage after CPB is caused by relatively large particulate or air emboli originating in the operative field[32, 37] during aortic manipulation or cannulation and on termination of bypass. The significance of macroembolism is indicated by the increased incidence of cerebral damage after "open-ventricle" procedures, especially if valvular calcification[37, 39] is present. The preponderance of right hemispheric stroke after "open" procedures also suggests embolism.[30, 32, 34, 46, 68] Presumably, emboli most frequently enter the first great vessel arising from the aorta.[32] The reported efficacy of thiopental prophylaxis during "open" procedures also supports an embolic cause,[37] since experimental data indicate that barbiturates protect the brain against focal,[69, 70] but not global,[71, 72] ischemia. Macroembolism might account for the association of brain damage with age. Atheromatous or calcific emboli might be more common in elderly patients with degenerative aortic disease.[38]

A combination of meticulous surgical technique and pharmacologic and/or hypothermic prophylaxis can probably reduce the incidence of macroembolic cerebral damage substantially.[37] This question is discussed in detail elsewhere in this monograph. The size of cerebral infarcts caused by macroembolic events occurring during aortic cannulation or manipulation also might be altered by variables such as anesthetic depth, temperature, acid–base management, perfusion flow rate, pulse wave pattern, and cerebral perfusion pressure during bypass.

SUMMARY AND RECOMMENDATIONS

Both anesthesia and hypothermia reduce $CMRO_2$. The combination of conventional high-dose narcotic-benzodiazepine anesthesia and moderate hypothermia (25° to 28° C) reduces $CMRO_2$ to 10 per cent of anticipated awake normothermic values during nonpulsatile CPB. A very small additional reduction in $CMRO_2$ can be achieved by abolition of electroencephalographic activity with thiopental or isoflurane. Such marked reduction in oxygen requirements may potentially protect the brain against ischemic insults during bypass. Temperature-related changes in $CMRO_2$ during bypass are consistent with a Q_{10} of approximately 2.5. Intravenous anesthetics preserve, while volatile anesthetics abolish, flow-metabolism coupling.

The CBF response to hypothermic bypass is profoundly affected by acid–base management. Alpha-stat acid–base management preserves flow-metabolism coupling and autoregulation, whereas pH-stat management causes pressure-dependent cerebral hyperperfusion. The practice of adding CO_2 to the oxygenator inflow during hypothermic bypass is intuitively objectionable because it apparently interferes with cerebrovascular homeostasis and is theoretically hazardous. Although outcome data are lacking, the ostensibly more physiologic alpha-stat pH management strategy appears preferable.

Nonpulsatile bypass in humans has been associated with $CMRO_2$ values that are 30 per cent to 40 per cent less than anticipated. In animals, pulsatile flow increases CBF in both normal and ischemic brain, compared with nonpulsatile flow. Further experiments in humans are needed. Currently the potential benefits of pulsation appear to outweigh the theoretical disadvantages.[73]

The range of cerebrovascular autoregulation during hypothermia is disputed. Although pooled data from clinical studies indicate a lower autoregulatory threshold of 20 to 30 mm Hg, other studies suggest a pressure-passive cerebral circulation when MAP is less than 50 mm Hg. Differences in temperature and depth of anesthesia may explain these contradictory results. In experiments in which flow was pressure-passive, increased O_2 extraction from arterial blood appeared to compensate for reduced cerebral oxygen delivery during hypotension, in the absence of cerebrovascular disease. Until prospective studies clearly define the autoregulatory threshold under various clinical circumstances, arterial pressure of less than 50 mm Hg should be regarded as a potential physiologic trespass, which may encroach on reserve capacity for cerebral oxygen delivery. In patients with cerebrovascular disease and/or hypertension, higher perfusion pressures may be required.

Perfusion flow rate is the major determinant of arterial pressure during bypass. In the absence of pharmacologic support, MAP is about 30 mm Hg when Q is 1 to 1.2 $l \cdot min^{-1} \cdot m^{-2}$ during profound (20° C) hypothermia. Lower flows and pressures have resulted in neurophysiologic deterioration in animal experiments. Flows of 1.5 to 1.6 $l \cdot min^{-1} \cdot m^{-2}$ are probably acceptable during moderate (25° to 28° C) hypothermia.

Retrospective analyses indicate that cerebral damage after bypass is often unrelated to the conduct of perfusion. Clearly, macroembolism accounts for a significant proportion of morbidity, especially after open-ventricle procedures. Similarly, episodes of hypotension and low cardiac output states that occur before or after bypass may cause global cerebral hypoperfusion.

The influence of perfusion-related variables such as Q, MAP, pulse wave pattern, and microembolism on the incidence and severity of perioperative brain damage has not been established. The consistent association of neurologic damage with patient age and duration of bypass suggests that global cerebral hypoperfusion and/or diffuse microembolism during bypass contributes to adverse neurologic outcome. Reports of "boundary-zone" infarction after bypass are also consistent with this hypothesis, as is evidence of reduced CBF and/or jugular venous desaturation associated with hypotension or nonpulsatile perfusion. Controversy over the importance of perfusion-related variables is entirely consequent on a lack of prospective clinical investigation. Prospective clinical trials that examine the influence of perfusion flow rate, perfusion pressure, pulsatile perfusion, oxygenator type, and arterial line microfiltration are urgently needed.

Our understanding of the influence of perfusion on cerebral physiology and function is rapidly advancing. Cardiac anesthesiologists will be better able to contribute to the management of perfusion if they have a solid working knowledge of this literature. The many controversies over appropriate management of bypass are likely to subside in the wake of well-conducted prospective clinical trials.

References

1. Shapiro HM: Anesthesia effects upon cerebral blood flow, cerebral metabolism, electroencephalogram, and evoked potentials. In Miller RD (ed): Anesthesia. New York, Churchill Livingstone, 1986, p 1249.
2. Lundar T, Frøysaker T, Lindegaard K-F, et al: Some observations on cerebral perfusion during cardiopulmonary bypass. Ann Thorac Surg 39:318, 1985.
3. Lundar T, Lindegaard K-F, Frøysaker T, et al: Cerebral perfusion during nonpulsatile cardiopulmonary bypass. Ann Thorac Surg 40:144, 1985.
4. Hägerdal M, Harp J, Nilsson L, Siesjö BK: The effect of induced hypothermia upon oxygen consumption in the rat brain. J Neurochem 24:311, 1975.
5. Wagerle LC, Orr JA, Shirer HW, et al: Cerebral vascular response to acute decreases in arterial Pa_{O_2}. J Cereb Blood Flow Metab 3:507, 1983.
6. Paulson OB, Parving H-H, Oleson J, et al: Influence of carbon monoxide and of hemodilution on cerebral blood flow and blood gases in man. J Appl Physiol 35:111, 1973.
7. Grubb RL, Raichle ME, Eichling JO, Ter-Pogossian MM: The effects of changes in Pa_{CO_2} on cerebral blood volume, blood flow, and vascular mean transit time. Stroke 5:630, 1974.
8. Henriksen L, Hjelms E, Lindeburgh T: Brain hyperperfusion during cardiac operations. Cerebral blood flow measured in man by intra-arterial injection of xenon 133: Evidence suggestive of intraoperative microembolism. J Thorac Cardiovasc Surg 86:202, 1983.
9. Henriksen L, Hjelms E: Cerebral blood flow during cardiopulmonary bypass in man: Effect of arterial filtration. Thorax 41:386, 1986.
10. Henriksen L: Brain luxury perfusion during cardiopulmonary bypass in humans. A study of the cerebral blood flow response to changes in CO_2, O_2, and blood pressure. J Cereb Blood Flow Metab 6:366, 1986.
11. Govier AV, Reves JG, McKay RD, et al: Factors and their influence on regional cerebral blood flow during nonpulsatile cardiopulmonary bypass. Ann Thorac Surg 38:592, 1984.
12. Prough DS, Stump DA, Roy RC, et al: Response of cerebral blood flow to changes in carbon dioxide tension during hypothermic cardiopulmonary bypass. Anesthesiology 64:576, 1986.
13. Feddersen K, Arén C, Nilsson NJ, Rådegran K: Cerebral blood flow and metabolism during cardiopulmonary bypass with special reference to effects of hypotension induced by prostacyclin. Ann Thorac Surg 41:395, 1986.

14. Murkin JM, Farrar JK, Tweed A, et al: Cerebral autoregulation and flow/metabolism coupling during cardiopulmonary bypass: The influence of Pa_{CO_2}. Anesth Analg 66:825, 1987.
15. Murkin JM, Farrar JK, Tweed WA, Guiraudon G: Cerebral blood flow, oxygen consumption and EEG during isoflurane anesthesia. Anesth Analg 65:S107, 1986.
16. Woodcock TE, Murkin JM, Farrar JK, et al: Pharmacologic EEG suppression during cardiopulmonary bypass: Cerebral hemodynamic and metabolic effects of thiopental or isoflurane during hypothermia and normothermia. Anesthesiology 67:218, 1987.
17. Murkin JM, Farrar K, Tweed AW, Guiraudon G: The influence of non-pulsatile normothermic perfusion on cerebral blood flow and metabolism. Anesth Analg 66:S125, 1987.
18. Kent B, Pierce EC II: Oxygen consumption during cardiopulmonary bypass in the uniformly cooled dog. J Appl Physiol 37:917, 1974.
19. Fox LS, Blackstone EH, Kirklin JW, et al: Relationship of whole body oxygen consumption to perfusion flow rate during hypothermic cardiopulmonary bypass. J Thorac Cardiovasc Surg 83:239, 1982.
20. Severinghaus JW: Blood gas claculator. J Appl Physiol 21:1108, 1966.
21. White FN, Weinstein Y: Carbon dioxide transport and acid–base balance during hypothermia. In Utley JR (ed): Pathophysiology and Techniques of Cardiopulmonary Bypass, Vol 2. Baltimore, Williams & Wilkins, 1983, p 40.
22. Rahn H, Reeves RB, Howell BJ: Hydrogen ion regulation, temperature, and evolution. Am Rev Respir Dis 112:165, 1975.
23. Reeves RB: The interaction of body temperature and acid–base balance in ectothermic vertebrates. Ann Rev Physiol 39:559, 1977.
24. Ellis RJ, Wisniewski A, Potts R, et al: Reduction of flow rate and arterial pressure at moderate hypothermia does not result in cerebral dysfunction. J Thorac Cardiovasc Surg 79:173, 1980.
25. Arén C, Badr G, Feddersen K, Rådegran K: Somatosensory evoked potentials and cerebral metabolism during cardiopulmonary bypass with special reference to hypotension induced by prostacyclin infusion. J Thorac Cardiovasc Surg 90:73, 1985.
26. Rebeyka IM, Coles JG, Wilson GJ, et al: The effect of low-flow cardiopulmonary bypass on cerebral function: An experimental and clinical study. Ann Thorac Surg 43:391, 1987.
27. Miyamoto K, Kawashima Y, Matsuda H, et al: Optimal perfusion flow rate for the brain during deep hypothermic cardiopulmonary bypass at 20° C: An experimental study. J Thorac Cardiovasc Surg 92:1065, 1986.
28. Sørensen HR, Husum B, Waaben J, et al: Brain microvascular function during cardiopulmonary bypass. J Thorac Cardiovasc Surg 94:727, 1987.
29. Tranmer BI, Gross CE, Kindt GW, Adey GR: Pulsatile versus nonpulsatile blood flow in the treatment of acute cerebral ischemia. Neurosurgery 19:724, 1986.
30. Sotaniemi KA, Juolasmaa A, Hokkanen ET: Neuropsychologic outcome after open-heart surgery. Arch Neurol 38:2, 1981.
31. Sotaniemi KA: Cerebral outcome after extracorporeal circulation: Comparison between prospective and retrospective examinations. Arch Neurol 40:75, 1983.
32. Slogoff S, Girgis KZ, Keats AS: Etiologic factors in neuropsychiatric complications associated with cardiopulmonary bypass. Anesth Analg 61:903, 1982.
33. Breuer AC, Furlan AJ, Hanson MR, et al: Central nervous system complications of coronary artery bypass graft surgery: Prospective analysis of 421 patients. Stroke 14:682, 1983.
34. Heikkinen L: Clinically significant neurological disorders following open-heart surgery. J Thorac Cardiovasc Surg 33:201, 1985.
35. Shaw PJ, Bates D, Cartlidge NEF, et al: Early neurological complications of coronary artery bypass surgery. Br Med J 291:1384, 1985.
36. Smith PLC, Treasure TT, Newman SP, et al: Cerebral consequences of cardiopulmonary bypass. Lancet 1:823, 1986.
37. Nussmeier NA, Arlund C, Slogoff S: Neuropsychiatric complications after cardiopulmonary bypass: Cerebral protection by a barbiturate. Anesthesiology 64:165, 1986.
38. Gardner TJ, Horneffer PJ, Manolio TA, et al: Stroke following coronary artery bypass grafting: A ten-year study. Ann Thorac Surg 40:574, 1985.

39. Åberg T, Kihlgren M: Effect of open heart surgery on intellectual function. Scand J Thorac Cardiovasc Surg 15 (Suppl) :1–63, 1974.
40. Åberg A, Kihlgren M: Cerebral protection during open-heart surgery. Thorax 32:525, 1977.
41. Arén C, Blomstrand C, Wikkelsö C, Rådegran K: Hypotension induced by prostacyclin treatment during cardiopulmonary bypass does not increase the risk of cerebral complications. J Thorac Cardiovasc Surg 88:748, 1984.
42. Kolkka R, Hilberman M: Neurologic dysfunction following cardiac operation with low-flow, low-pressure cardiopulmonary bypass. J Thorac Cardiovasc Surg 79:432, 1980.
43. Gilman S: Cerebral disorders after open-heart operations. N Engl J Med 272:489, 1965.
44. Lee WH Jr, Brady MP, Rowe JM, Miller WC: Effects of extracorporeal circulation upon behavior, personality, and brain function. II. Hemodynamic, metabolic and psychometric correlations. Ann Surg 173:1013, 1971.
45. Tufo HM, Ostfeld AM, Shekelle R: Central nervous system dysfunction following open-heart surgery. JAMA 212:1333, 1970.
46. Branthwaite MA: Neurological damage related to open-heart surgery. A clinical survey. Thorax 27:748, 1972.
47. Branthwaite MA: Prevention of neurological damage during open-heart surgery. Thorax 30:258, 1975.
48. Stockard JJ, Bickford RG, Schauble JF: Pressure-dependent cerebral ischemia during cardiopulmonary bypass. Neurology 23:521, 1973.
49. Gonzáàlez–Scareno F, Hurtig HI: Neurologic complications of coronary artery bypass grafting: Case-control study. Neurology (NY) 31:1032, 1981.
50. Rabiner CJ, Willner AE, Fishman J: Psychiatric complications following coronary bypass surgery. J Nerv Ment Dis 160:342, 1975.
51. Brierley JB, Prior PF, Calverley J, et al: The pathogenesis of ischemic neuronal damage along the cerebral arterial boundary zones in papio anubis. Brain 103:929, 1980.
52. Malone M, Prior P, Scholtz CL: Brain damage after cardiopulmonary by-pass: Correlations between neurophysiological and neuropathological findings. J Neurol Neurosurg Psychiatry 44:924, 1981.
53. Taugher PJ: Visual loss after cardiopulmonary bypass. Am J Ophthalmol 81:280, 1976.
54. Gravlee GP, Hudspeth AS, Toole JF: Bilateral brachial paralysis from watershed infarction after coronary artery bypass. J Thorac Cardiovasc Surg 88:742, 1984.
55. Russell RWR, Bharucha N: The recognition and prevention of border zone cerebral ischaemia during cardiac surgery. Q J Med 47:303, 1978.
56. Gallagher EG, Pearson DT: Ultrasonic identification of sources of gaseous microemboli during open heart surgery. Thorax 28:295, 1973.
57. Hatteland K, Pedersen T, Semb BKH: Comparison of bubble release from various types of oxygenators. Scand J Thorac Cardiovasc Surg 19:125, 1985.
58. Loop FD, Szabo J, Rowlinson RD, Urbanek K: Events related to microembolism during extracorporeal perfusion in man: Effectiveness of in-line filtration recorded by ultrasound. Ann Thorac Surg 21:412, 1976.
59. Lee WH, Krumhaar K, Fonkalsrud EW, et al: Denaturation of plasma proteins as a cause of morbidity and death after intracardiac operations. Surgery 50:29, 1961.
60. Hill JD, Aguilar MJ, Baranco A, et al: Neuropathological manifestations of cardiac surgery. Ann Thorac Surg 7:409, 1969.
61. Solis RT, Kennedy PS, Beall AC Jr, et al: Cardiopulmonary bypass. Microembolization and platelet aggregation. Circulation 52:103, 1975.
62. Chenoweth DE, Cooper SW, Hugli TE, et al: Complement activation during cardiopulmonary bypass. Evidence for generation of C3a and C5a anaphylatoxins. N Engl J Med 304:497, 1981.
63. Van Oeveren A, Kazatchkine MD, Descamps–Latscha B, et al: Deleterious effects of cardiopulmonary bypass: A prospective study of bubble versus membrane oxygenation. J Thorac Cardiovasc Surg 89:888, 1985.
64. Calafiore AM, Glieca F, Marchesani F, et al: A comparative clinical assessment of a hollow-fibre membrane oxygenator (Capiox II) and a bubble oxygenator (Harvey 1500). J Thorac Cardiovasc Surg 28:633, 1987.
65. Cavarocchi NC, Pluth JR, Schaff HV, et al: Complement activation during cardiopul-

monary bypass: Comparison of a bubble and membrane oxygenators. J Thorac Cardiovasc Surg 91:252, 1968.

66. Padayachee TS, Parsons S, Theobold R, et al: The detection of microemboli in the middle cerebral artery during cardiopulmonary bypass: A transcranial Doppler ultrasound investigation using membrane and bubble oxygenators. Ann Thorac Surg 88:298, 1987.

67. Aris A, Solanes H, Cámara ML, et al: Arterial line filtration during cardiopulmonary bypass. Neurologic, neuropsychologic and hematologic studies. J Thorac Cardiovasc Surg 91:526, 1986.

68. Björk VO, Ivert T: Early and late neurological complications after prosthetic heart valve replacement. In Becker R, et al (eds): Psychopathological and Neurological Dysfunctions Following Open-Heart Surgery. Heidelberg, Springer-Verlag, 1982, p 3.

69. Smith AL, Hoff JT, Nielson SL, Larson CP: Barbiturate protection in acute focal cerebral ischemia. Stroke 5:127, 1974.

70. Michenfelder JD, Milde JH, Sunkt TM Jr: Cerebral protection by barbiturate anesthesia. Arch Neurol 33:345, 1976.

71. Steen PA, Milde JH, Michenfelder JD: No barbiturate protection in a dog model of complete cerebral ischemia. Ann Neurol 5:343, 1979.

72. Gisvold SE, Safar P, Hendricks HHL, et al: Thiopental treatment after global brain ischemia in pigtailed monkeys. Anesthesiology 60:88, 1984.

73. Hickey PR, Buckley MJ, Philbin DM: Pulsatile and nonpulsatile cardiopulmonary bypass: Review of counterproductive controversy. Ann Thorac Surg 36:720, 1983.

CHAPTER 3

CENTRAL NERVOUS SYSTEM COMPLICATIONS AFTER CARDIOPULMONARY BYPASS

ANN V. GOVIER

The development of cardiopulmonary bypass (CPB) has been essential to many remarkable improvements in the surgical management of heart disease. The number of cardiac operations that require CPB has steadily increased over the past 30 years. In North America alone an estimated 200,000 such surgeries are performed each year.[1] Although advances in surgical technique, anesthetic management, and the extracorporeal apparatus have substantially reduced the morbidity and mortality related to CPB, unpredictable transient and permanent central nervous system (CNS) complications continue to occur. The exact causes of these CNS injuries, which become apparent after otherwise uncomplicated heart surgery, are still not understood. Numerous studies[2-11] have shown that the morbidity and mortality associated with the surgical management of coronary artery disease have been decreasing. Those who have studied these declines[2, 4-6, 8-11] suggest that the decreased surgical risk results from (a) better preoperative stabilization of critically ill patients; (b) improved perioperative patient management (especially upgraded surgical and anesthetic techniques, including better intraoperative myocardial protection); and (c) intensive postoperative care.

A careful review of morbidity trends from the early 1970's to the early 1980's reveals that the morbidity associated with perioperative myocardial infarction, reoperation for bleeding, respiratory insufficiency, gastrointestinal bleeding, and other nonneurologic complications has declined. However, the morbidity associated with neurologic complications has not satisfactorily declined.[2, 5, 11] In a recent review of the trends in surgical mortality from 1970 to 1980 by Cosgrove et al.,[5] neurologic deficits were the second most frequent cause of death (after cardiac complications) in patients undergoing primary myocardial revasculari-

TABLE 3–1. STUDIES REPORTING INCIDENCE OF CEREBRAL DYSFUNCTION AFTER OPEN HEART OPERATIONS[27]

Reference	No. of Patients	Perspective	Type of Observation	Incidence Transient	Incidence Persistent	Closed or Open Operation	Prime
Ehrenhaft et al., 1961[12]	244	R	C	7.0	1.6	I	NR
Gillman, 1965[13]	35	P	C + P	34.0	23.0	I	NR
Kornfeld et al., 1965[14]	78	P	C + P	38.0	NR	I	NR
Gilberstadt & Sako, 1967[15]	53	P	C + P	13.0	13.0	I	NR
Tufo et al., 1970[16]	85	P	C + P	44.0	15.0	I	B
Lee et al., 1971[17]	71	P	C + P	31.0	NR	I	B
Branthwaite, 1972[18]	417	R	C	19.2	9.1	I	B
Stockard et al., 1973[19]	25	P	C	36.0	12.1	I + E	NR
Branthwaite, 1975[20]	528	R	C	7.4	4.8	I + E	B
Åberg & Kihlgren, 1977[21]	223	P	C + P	8.5	NR	I + E	B + C
Ellis et al., 1980[22]	30	P	C + P	0.0	0.0	E	C
Breuer et al., 1981[23]	418	R	C	16.0	NR	E	NR
Kolka & Hilberman, 1980[24]	204	P	C + P	40.0	17.2	I + E	C
Turnipseed et al., 1980[25]	170	R	C	NR	5.3	E	C
Slogoff et al., 1982[26]	204	P	C + P	16.2	6.4	I + E	C
Govier et al., 1984[27]	17	P	C + P	0	0	E	C

Perspective, retrospective (R) or prospective (P); type of observations, clinical (C) or psychometric (P); closed or open operation, intracardiac (I) or extracardiac (E); prime, blood (B) or crystalloid (C); NR, not reported.

zation. Although the relative percentage of deaths owing to cardiac causes has decreased from the early 1970's to the 1980's, "other causes of death [have relatively] increased, the most notable being neurological deficits, which [have] increased from 7.2% to 19.6%."[5]

This chapter describes the CNS complications of cardiac surgery, including fatal cerebral damage, stroke, and neuropsychologic dysfunction. Possible causes of this cerebral damage are reviewed. The chapter concludes with a discussion of therapies currently proposed and/or under evaluation for cerebral protection.

CENTRAL NERVOUS SYSTEM COMPLICATIONS

The reported incidence of neurologic and/or neuropsychologic dysfunction after cardiac operations using CPB ranges from 0 per cent to 40 per cent (Table 3–1).[12–27] This variation is probably as much a result of study techniques and data collection as it is of actual variations in that which was measured. For example, Slogoff et al.,[26] have shown that the incidence reported is influenced by the study design (retrospective versus prospective analysis), the sensitivity and specificity of the study methodology, and the type of cardiac surgery. Sotaniemi[28] found that patients retrospectively analyzed by nonneurologists had a 6 per cent incidence of postoperative cerebral abnormalities, whereas patients examined prospectively by neurologists had a 35 per cent incidence of damage.

Fatal Cerebal Damage

In 1960 Bjork and Hultquist[29] published an early study of the cerebral pathology of fatal post-CPB brain damage. Five of the 11 fatalities after extracorporeal circulation died of brain damage. They were children (under 6 years of age) who had been subjected to deep hypothermia (5–16° C). The authors believed that the exposure to deep hypothermia caused the fatal cerebral injury.

In 1963 Brierley[30] also reported neuropathologic findings for 11 patients who died within 2 weeks of heart surgery. Nine of the patients underwent CPB. Two patients underwent deliberate circulatory arrest under moderate hypothermia without the use of CPB. Cortical damage occurred predominantly in the posterior brain, with sparing of the brain stem. The "typical" neuropathologic picture of cerebral anoxia was present in only one CPB case, and it was attributed to a postoperative cardiac arrest at normal body temperature. Based on the neuropathologic findings in these 11 cases, Brierley[30] concluded that air embolism and hypotension associated with severely reduced cerebral blood flow (CBF) were the principal causes of the neuropathologic changes.

TABLE 3–2. SUMMARY OF RECENT DATA ON CNS COMPLICATIONS OF OPEN HEART SURGERY[45]

Authors	Year*	Study Design	Type of OHS	No. of Patients	Percentage with CNS Deficit		Method of Ascertainment
					Focal Infarct	Encephalopathy	
Hill JD et al.[35]	1968	Pathologic analysis autopsy cases	Mixture	133	** (fat emboli in 62% brains, non-fat emboli in 31% brains)	**	Pathologic analysis of brains
Heller SS et al.[36]	1969	Prospective	Mixture	100	** (24% had postop delirium)	9%	Psychiatric interview, psychologic testing
Javid H et al.[37]	1969	Prospective	Mixture	100	13+%	35%	Clinical exam, psychologic testing
Tufo HM et al.[16]	1969	Prospective	Mixture	100	13+%	43%	Clinical exam, psychologic testing
Branthwaite MA[18]	1970	Retrospective, % prospective	Mixture	417	9.4%	10.1%	Chart review, clinical exam
Hansotia P et al.[38]	1972	Prospective	Mixture	177	** (51% with persistently abnormal EEG at discharge. Includes 11 patients who died.)	**	Serial EEG
Cannom DS et al.[39]	1972	Retrospective	Mixture	400	1%∧	**	Chart review
Hutchinson JE et al.[6]	1972	Retrospective	CABG alone	376	0.3%∧	**	Chart review

Study	Year	Design	Population	N			Method
Branthwaite MA[40]	1973	Prospective	Mixture	140	**	** (7.1% had clinical neurologic damage)	Intraoperative use of cerebral function monitor
Branthwaite MA[20]	1973	Retrospective	Mixture	538	3%	4.8%	Chart review
Hodgman JR et al.[41]	1974	Retrospective	Mixture	100	**	** (20% has minor psychiatric problems)/\	Chart review
Kolkka R et al.[24]	1977	Prospective	Mixture	204	2.9%	17.2%	Clinical exam
Lee MC et al.[42]	1978	Retrospective	Mixture	943	0.7%	**	Chart review
Gonzalez-Scarano F et al.[43]	1978	Retrospective case-control	CABG alone	1427	1%	0.4%	Chart review
Loop FD et al.[11]	1978	Retrospective	CABG alone	8741	1.3%–2%/\	**	Chart review, computerized cardiovascular info registry
Muraoka R et al.[44]	1979	Prospective	Congenital heart disease	57	0% (10.5% had persistent CT scan changes)	0%	Chart review
Turnipseed WD et al.[25]	1979	Prospective	CABG alone	170	4.7%	**	Clinical exam
Breuer AC et al.[45]	1980	Prospective	CABG alone	421	5.2% (total) 2% (severe)	11.6%	Clinical exam
Shaw et al.[33]	1984	Prospective	CABG alone	312	5%	3% (prolonged depression) 1% (psychosis)	Clinical exam, psychologic testing

*Last year patients in study underwent surgery reflecting technology of that time (i.e., not year study published).

/\These retrospective studies are largely devoted to analyses of nonneurologic issues and complications and mention CNS dysfunction.

**No clinical examination data available.

Aguilar et al.[31] reported relevant neuropathologic abnormalities in 85 per cent of 206 patients who died after open heart surgery. The principal lesions were focal hemorrhages, acute neuronal necroses, and emboli. The presence of nonfat emboli was positively correlated with the duration of extracorporeal circulation. In Sotaniemi's[32] prospective study of 100 patients undergoing cardiac valve replacement, two patients (2 per cent mortality) died within 4 days of surgery without regaining consciousness. Brain damage was the principal cause of death as evidenced by multiple small hemorrhages and acute ischemic neuronal damage in the cerebral hemispheres, brain stem, and cerebellum.

Recent studies have indicated that the absolute incidence of fatal cerebral injury after cardiac surgery is decreasing.[23, 33] In a prospective study (January through December 1980) of 531 cardiac operations at the Cleveland Clinic, death associated with severe CNS deficit occurred in 3 of 418 patients (0.7 per cent).[23] In a prospective study by Shaw et al.[33] of 312 patients having coronary artery bypass graft (CABG) surgery, fatal cerebral hypoxic damage occurred in only 1 patient (0.3 per cent).

Stroke

A stroke is a focal CNS deficit that occurs relatively suddenly and lasts for more than 24 hours.[34] Reported frequencies of this focal cerebral infarction after heart surgery vary from 0 per cent to more than 13 per cent (Table 3–2).[6, 11, 16, 18, 20, 24, 25, 33, 35–45] Breuer et al.[45] emphasize that the reported frequency of focal infarct is directly influenced by the "study design, the method of [the infarct's] ascertainment, the personnel conducting the neurological assessment, the types of heart procedures being evaluated, and the differences in patient selection and surgical technique [between] different institutions."

Controversy exists over whether there may be a higher incidence of stroke after intracardiac heart operations (such as valvular surgery) than after CABG and other extracardiac surgeries. In a prospective study by Sotaniemi[32] of 100 patients undergoing open heart operations for valve replacement, 24 were found to have at least transient postoperative hemiparesis. In 1985 Heikkinen et al.[46] reported that every case they found of postsurgical hemiplegia or hemiparesis was associated with valve replacement (either single or multivalve procedures). In contrast, Furlan and Breuer[47] reported that the 5 per cent stroke incidence associated with CABG surgery (421 patients) did not significantly differ (6 per cent) from that of other forms of cardiac surgery (99 patients). In a prospective study Breuer et al.[48] compared the postoperative stroke frequency of 421 patients who underwent only CABG with that of 80 patients who underwent valve replacement both with and without concomitant CABG. Although exposing the left heart chamber during valve surgery theoretically might have increased the risk of embolism, there was no significant difference in stroke frequency associated with CABG (5.2 per cent) and valve (7.5 per cent) surgery. Breuer et al.[48] concluded that operative techniques, such as aortic cross-clamping, used in both CABG and valvular surgery may be important in generating embolic debris, which may cause stroke in this setting.

Several investigators[5, 18, 49–53] have reported that elderly patients have a significantly greater incidence of postoperative strokes than do younger patients. Gardner et al.[49] concluded that "elderly patients who have preexisting vascular disease or who require (an) extensive revascularization procedure, or who have severe atherosclerosis of the ascending aorta have a significantly increased risk of postoperative stroke." Cosgrove et al.[5] theorized that the increased incidence of cerebrovascular accidents (strokes) with advanced age "probably [results from] the increased potential for aortic atherosclerosis with embolization and extracranial cerebral vascular disease in older patients."

Breuer et al.[54] have reported that left ventricular thrombi significantly increase the risk of stroke during heart surgery. A retrospective analysis of 28,831 cardiac catheterizations from 1976 to 1980 identified 403 patients (1.4 per cent) who had definite left ventricular intraluminal filling defects that were interpreted as mural thrombi. One hundred fifty-five (38 per cent) of these 403 patients had subsequent heart surgery. Fifteen strokes occurred in the immediate postoperative period—a stroke frequency of 9.6 per cent. This was more than four times the postoperative serious stroke frequency (2 per cent) found in patients without left ventricular thrombi in a prospective study at the Cleveland Clinic.[45]

Controversy exists as to whether carotid stenosis or history of transient cerebral ischemia is associated with an increased incidence of subsequent stroke.[25, 55–57] Barnes et al.[55] and Turnipseed et al.[25] could not relate the incidence of perioperative strokes to the presence of high-grade carotid stenoses. Turnipseed et al.[25] found no direct relation between a carotid bruit or the severity of preexisting carotid artery disease and the incidence of perioperative strokes in patients undergoing either elective CABG or peripheral vascular reconstructive surgery. Significantly, that study included both patients with antecedent neurologic symptoms and asymptomatic patients.

NEUROPSYCHOLOGIC DYSFUNCTION

Delirium and Organic Brain Syndrome

Numerous studies[14, 15, 58–65] have reported various types and incidences of neuropsychologic dysfunction after cardiac surgery. Gotze et al.[66] have published an excellent review and survey of these studies. For several reasons cross-comparison of the data and results from these studies is difficult. First, most reported a variety of psychiatric symptoms, ranging from delirium to depression, without a uniform system of classification. Second, the design of the studies varied greatly. Different psychometric tests were used that were not always administered by appropriately trained individuals. The timing and details of postoperative assessments varied. Third, the patients' ages and socioeconomic levels, which may affect test performance, were not always recorded. Finally, the actual incidence and magnitude of neuropsychologic impairment may be decreasing.

Edgerton and Kay[58] reported high incidences of delirium after cardiotomy as early as 1964. In 1970 Heller et al.[36] attempted to classify the neuropsychologic complications associated with heart surgery into two categories. The first were those complications that became apparent when the patient first awoke from anesthesia. These were labeled early postoperative "organic brain syndrome." Mildly affected patients might incorrectly identify the day, date, or year. Those more severely affected were disoriented with respect to person and place. The most severely affected patients were comatose. Some died without regaining consciousness. Their second category of complications was composed of patients who had a lucid interval of 2 to 5 days followed by the onset of hallucinations and delusions. This category was labeled "postcardiotomy delirium." These patients had difficulty distinguishing between dreams and reality. Severe disorientation developed, especially at night. Patients often reported experiencing frightening hallucinatory episodes.

Many studies, including that of Heller et al.,[36] have attempted to identify the cause(s) of neuropsychologic dysfunction (either delirium or organic brain syndrome) by examining a wide variety of preoperative, intraoperative, and postoperative factors.

Preoperative Factors Related to Neuropsychologic Dysfunction

Heller et al.[36] reported that post-CPB organic brain syndrome and delirium were related to advancing age. This has been confirmed by a number of others.[37, 58, 59, 65, 67] Savageau et al.[65] reported that patients older than 60 performed significantly worse postoperatively on a variety of neuropsychologic tests than did younger patients.

Kornfeld et al.,[14] Heller et al.,[36] Blanchy and Starr,[59] and Edgerton and Kay[58] reported that development of neuropsychologic dysfunction was related to the nature of the patient's heart disease (i.e., acquired heart disease or congenital heart disease [CHD]). Kornfeld et al.[14] reported that acute post-CPB organic psychosis did not occur in any of the 20 children in their series. Heller et al.[36] reported that while delirium occurred in 26 per cent of the patients with acquired heart disease, it occurred in only 8 per cent of those with CHD. Blanchy and Starr[59] also found that those with CHD had a lower incidence of delirium. They pointed out, however, that these patients were younger and generally less ill preoperatively than other cardiac patients.

A variety of other preoperative factors have been found to correlate positively with increased incidence of neuropsychologic dysfunction. A number of authors have reported that the preoperative severity of illness or the patient's physical incapacity significantly increased the incidence of delirium or early organic brain syndrome.[14, 36, 59] Other investigators[59, 61] have reported a correlation between preoperative psychologic factors and delirium after open heart surgery. Branthwaite[20] and Javid et al.[37] found an increased incidence of neuropsychologic dysfunction in patients who had a preoperative history of neurologic or cerebral vascular abnormalities. Heller et al.[36] found that patients who received minor tranquilizers on a regular basis before surgery had an increased incidence of postoperative delirium.

Perioperative Factors Related to Neuropsychologic Dysfunction

Factors related to the operative procedure itself have been reported to correlate positively with neuropsychologic disorders. Heller et al.,[36] Blanchy and Starr,[59] and Kornfeld et al.[14] reported a higher incidence of postoperative delirium in patients who had multiple-valve surgical procedures compared with those who had single-valve procedures, possibly because multiple-valve procedures often involve longer bypass times. A number of investigators have reported that the incidence and severity of neuropsychologic dysfunction increase with prolonged bypass time— regardless of the surgical procedure.[15, 37, 65, 68–70] Earlier studies reported that postoperative delirium occurred after CABG surgery in up to 28 per cent of patients, a rate comparable to that reported for patients having intracardiac surgery.[64] However, in a recent study (1987) by Calabrese et al.,[63] postoperative delirium was found to follow myocardial revascularization less frequently than reported for other cardiac surgeries. In this study only four CABG patients (6.8 per cent) showed transient signs of confusion in the intensive care unit the day after surgery. None of the 59 CABG patients exhibited signs of delirium by the 6th day.

Postoperative Factors Related to Neuropsychologic Dysfunction

Heller et al.[36] found a significantly increased incidence of delirium and early organic brain syndrome in patients who were severely ill postoperatively. Kornfeld et al.[64] found that the only variable that correlated positively with delirium after CABG surgery was severity of postoperative illness. Other postoperative factors that have been correlated with neuropsychologic dysfunction include sleep deprivation,[14, 36, 58] low cardiac output,[62, 64] postoperative dehydration,[58] electrolyte abnormalities,[58, 65] abnormal sensory input,[14, 15, 58] arrhythmias,[71] acute renal shutdown,[59] propranolol administration,[72] and depression.[65, 73]

Intellectual/Cognitive Changes

Despite improvements in surgical, anesthetic, and perfusion techniques, neuropsychologic dysfunction remains a significant complication of heart surgery. Although most neuropsychologic abnormalities are transient and may have little long-term significance, a small percentage of patients do suffer permanent disabilities.[74] Neuropsychologic testing is believed to be the best way to quantitatively assess postoperative cognitive function.[75] Such testing was first used by Priest et al.[76] in 1957 to assess changes in intellectual function after non-CPB heart surgery. They found that performance on psychologic tests of organic function worsened after closed mitral commissurotomy and that this effect lasted as long as 6 months. In 1982 Åberg et al.[77] reported that 33 of 36 patients after undergoing cardiac surgery with CPB, who showed decreased intellectual function as measured by psychometric testing, had adenylate kinase in their cerebrospinal fluid—a biochemical marker of brain damage.

Although it is difficult to compare results from the various studies of postoperative cognitive dysfunction, in general, the earlier and more extensively the patients were tested, the higher the incidence and severity of the observed deficits.[34] A number of investigators[22, 34, 68, 73] have shown that early intellectual dysfunction usually resolves in the first few months after cardiac surgery. Ellis et al.[22] assessed 30 patients undergoing CABG surgery and found that 75 per cent had significantly impaired cognitive function early after the operation. Later, at 1 month, 25 of the 30 patients had no clinically measurable cognitive function impairment, and after 6 months none had impaired performance. Savageau et al.[73] neuropsychologically tested 245 patients both before and 6 months after CPB. Twenty-eight per cent were cognitively impaired in the early postoperative period, but only 5 per cent had persistent postoperative score deterioration after 6 months. In this study the functional decrement observed after 6 months seemed to be associated with the estimated loss of greater than 3,000 ml of blood during the operation but was also associated with perioperative administration of propranolol. In 1981 Sotaniemi et al.[68] showed that 56.5 per cent of patients who had clinical evidence of actual cerebral complications plus 7.7 per cent of those without were neuropsychologically impaired for up to 2 months after operations for valvular disease.

Other authors have questioned whether intellectual dysfunction actually resolves within 3 to 6 months of the operation. They have speculated that test score improvement results from practice rather than from actual cognitive improvement. Frank et al.[78] evaluated 98 patients by psychologic testing before heart surgery. Approximately half were retested 6 months after the operation. Their data indicated that although intelligence test scores 6 months postoperatively were higher on the average, improvement appeared to result primarily from practice. The effect of practice could be only partially controlled by using different tests. Juolasmaa et al.[79] and Åberg[80] also concluded that familiarity with the test situation and practice explained improved test results.

A number of studies[75, 80, 81] have indicated that general surgical operations with conventional anesthesia produce fewer changes in cognitive function than do cardiac operations. Raymond et al.[81] found significant deterioration in psychometric test performance in patients undergoing CABG surgery, but not in patients who had major peripheral vascular surgery of comparable duration. Over a 2-year period, Åberg[80] compared psychometric test results of 144 patients who underwent cardiac surgery with CPB with those of 53 general thoracic surgery patients. Overall, the test results of the general thoracic surgery group stayed at the preoperative level or actually improved. The cardiac surgery patients showed marked impairment of intellectual function. Åberg[80] concluded that extracorporeal circulation brings about impairment in intellectual function and that such impairment probably indicates cerebral injury. By contrast, in a prospective study, Smith et al.[69] found similar neuropsychologic deficits in patients undergoing thoracic or major vascular surgery. This study casts doubt on the theory that it is exclusively CPB that generates these changes.

In a recent study (1987) by Calabrese et al.,[63] cognitive function was prospectively studied in 59 patients undergoing CABG. A variety of neuropsychologic tests showed subtle but significant postoperative (day 6) cognitive deficits in the younger as well as older patients. Their data suggest that duration of anesthesia and of bypass, hematocrit and body temperature during bypass, and perfusion pressure time below 50 mm Hg do not account for these deficits.

Despite significant advances in CPB since its first use, the physiologic environment it creates is artificial and imperfect. There is still a disturbing incidence of cerebral dysfunction after heart surgery. These cognitive disorders are often subtle or even nearly asymptomatic and are often not severe enough to impair the great majority of survivors.[15, 75] However, as stated by Åberg and Kihlgren,[21] "there is still . . . a definite incidence of debilitating cerebral complications and of subclinical degrees of brain damage. These must be abolished."

POSSIBLE CAUSES OF CEREBRAL DAMAGE

Clinical and laboratory research have implicated three major causes of cerebral injury after heart surgery: microembolization, macroembolization, and inadequate cerebral perfusion.

Microembolization

Microembolization during CPB has been well documented and is regarded by many as a major cause of postoperative cerebral dysfunction and damage.[20, 21, 44, 82–87] Various types of microemboli are formed during CPB (Table 3–3).[88] All patients have microemboli that can be detected in the arterial inflow line during CPB.[88] Many solid microemboli are platelet and leukocyte aggregates that are formed and stored in bank blood and are resistant to deaggregation.[85, 89] Platelet and fibrin microaggregates can be formed during CPB despite apparently adequate heparinization.[34] The extracorporeal circulation (ECC) equipment itself may generate particulate matter such as plastic fragments.[34, 72, 88] In the past, antifoam chemicals in the pump oxygenator have been reported to generate silicon microemboli.[90, 91] Silicon emboli were usually spread throughout the body and were clinically manifested primarily in the brain (disturbance of sensorium), kidneys (hematuria), and eyes (retinal hemorrhage).[92] Modern equipment has eliminated this problem.

The pump oxygenator may also generate gaseous emboli. These have been detected by various means, including echo ultrasound[83, 84] and transesophageal echocardiograpy.[87] Microemboli of oxygen can arise during the oxygenation of the blood.[88, 93] Air embolism can result from incomplete defoaming of the blood in bubble oxygenators.[94] Microbubbles of dissolved gases may form if too great a temperature differential is established between the blood and heat exchanger,[88] especially during attempts at rapid rewarming. Design flaws in the cardiotomy suction have been sources of emboli during CPB.[94, 95] Microemboli may also arise from residual air left in the heart during the surgical procedure.[96, 97] Fat

TABLE 3–3. TYPES OF MICROEMBOLI FORMED DURING CPB[88]

Platelet	Lipid droplets
Leukocyte	Antifoam particles
Protein	Particulate matter
Calcium particles	Air
Muscle fragments	Oxygen

emboli suctioned from the operative site have been identified as a source of microemboli.[35] Hill et al.[35] reported fat emboli in the brains of 80 per cent of the heart surgery cases autopsied.

A number of studies[44, 83, 84, 86, 94, 98, 99] have revealed that arterial inflow line filters in the CPB circuit will reduce the number of microemboli and possibly decrease the incidence and extent of cerebral injury. Laboratory and clinical research must continue in order to provide additional knowledge of how microemboli are produced. This will lead to further reductions in the morbidity and mortality from cerebral complications of cardiac surgery. The extensive chapter by Fish[88] on microembolization, its cause and prevention, is recommended for a detailed review of this topic.

Macroembolization

Over the past two decades evidence has been accumulating that macroemboli from the surgical field are one of the most common causes of cerebral dysfunction after cardiac surgery.[13, 21, 23, 24, 26, 32, 43, 45, 53, 82, 87, 100–103] Massive air embolism, although rare during heart surgery, can lead to devastating neurologic complications. Massive air embolism during CPB resulted in instantaneous death in 4 of the 13 cases reviewed by Mills and Ochsner.[104] Possible causes of air embolism are listed in Table 3–4.[104] Various investigators[87, 93, 97] have shown that air embolism is more common during open-chamber operations (valvular surgery, ventricular aneurysm resection, or closure of a septal defect) than during CABG surgery. Air can be trapped in numerous locations within the heart: "atrial, ventricular or aortic cul-de-sacs, such as the left atrial appendage, the left ventricular apex between the chordae tendinae, the crevices between the papillary muscles, within the irregularities of the trabeculae carnae, and beneath the mural leaflet of the mitral valve."[105]

Large plaque debris from heart valves and vegetations on the valves themselves are additional sources of macroemboli.[13] This may be the

TABLE 3–4. CAUSES OF AIR EMBOLISM[104]

Inattention to oxygenator blood level
Unexpected resumption of heartbeat
Reversal of vent or perfusion lines in pump head
Pressurized cardiotomy reservoir
Opening a beating heart
Clotted oxygenator
Runaway pump head
Kink in arterial line proximal to pump head
Break in integrity of lines or oxygenator
Detachment of oxygenator during perfusion
Faulty technique during circulatory arrest
Unnoticed rotation of arterial pump head

reason that numerous investigators have shown greater incidence of severe neurologic deficits after valve replacement. These operations also have a significant influence on intellectual function.[13, 21, 26, 32, 100] According to Mills and Ochsner,[104] "non-fatal cerebral air injury may result in prolonged convalescence, yet complete recovery, whereas embolism from debris or clot . . . offers a poor prognosis."

The release of thrombi from the atrium or ventricle during surgery, or from the vein grafts or aortic sutures postoperatively, has been shown to lead to severe neurologic complications, including death.[23, 106, 107] During a 4-year period (1976–1980) at the Cleveland Clinic, 159 patients who had left ventricular intraluminal filling defects interpreted as mural thrombi underwent heart surgery.[54] Fifteen patients had strokes in the immediate postoperative period, a stroke frequency of 9.6 per cent (retrospective analysis). This was more than four times this institution's normal postoperative serious stroke rate (2 per cent as determined in a recent prospective study of 421 patients who did not have left ventricular mural thrombi).[45]

Atheromatous debris (e.g., calcific plaque or cholesterol) may be released by cannulation, cross-clamping, or decannulation of the ascending aorta. This material can also cause severe neurologic damage.[108] Martin and Hashimoto[101] reported a 3.2 per cent stroke incidence in a retrospective review of 253 CABG patients. They noted that all intraoperative strokes occurred in patients who had undergone femoral cannulation. Thus, in addition to the manipulation of the ascending aorta, the cannulation site may be a source of embolic material.

Identifying the sources of and preventing macroembolization are critical if the neurologic complications associated with cardiac surgery are to be eliminated. A detailed review of macroembolization, its prevention, and outcome modification may be found in Nussmeier and McDermott's recent review.[105]

Inadequate Cerebral Perfusion

The cause of inadequate cerebral perfusion pressure and the pathogenesis of related cerebral damage after CPB have been discussed by numerous authors.[12, 13, 17, 30, 42, 43, 90, 109–111] They have concluded that inadequate cerebral perfusion pressure can result from low mean arterial pressure (MAP), low perfusion flow, incorrect cannula placement, or extracranial/intracranial arterial occlusive disease.

Considerable controversy exists over the appropriate arterial blood pressure and its influence, if any, on CBF during each phase of CPB. Early studies[16, 37, 42] indicated that patients who had low arterial pressures during CPB had increased incidence of cerebral complications. Tufo et al.[16] in 1970 and Stockard et al.[112] in 1974 concluded that MAP should be maintained at greater than 50 mm Hg to avoid the postoperative cerebral dysfunction that they contended resulted from inadequate CBF. According to Tufo et al.,[16] "when MAP fell below 40 mm Hg there was a three-fold increase in the occurrence of cerebral damage over that observed if MAP remained above 60 mm Hg."

In contrast, Kolkka and Hilberman[24] prospectively studied 204 patients who underwent cardiac operations with hypothermic CPB and found no correlation between perfusion pressure and postoperative neurologic dysfunction. Their study suggested that "perfusion pressure, per se, is not the major determinant of postoperative cerebral dysfunction in an orderly operative procedure."[24] Sotaniemi et al,[68] in a study of 49 patients, documented episodes wherein the MAP ranged between 40 and 55 mm Hg for up to 25 minutes. This perfusion pressure was not found to produce any clinical, neuropsychologic, or quantitative electroencephalographic (EEG) consequences. They concluded that the effects of hypotension were dependent on other, coincidental factors. In 1980 Sotaniemi,[32] in a retrospective study of 100 patients who underwent valve replacement surgery, found that neither the degree nor the duration of moderate hypotension was significant in the cause of postoperative cerebral disorders. Slogoff et al.,[26] in a prospective study of 240 patients, were also unable to confirm any relation between postoperative cerebral dysfunction and perfusion pressures of less than 50 mm Hg during hypothermic CPB. In a combined prospective (364 patients) and retrospective (151 patients) study, Heikkinen[113] found no relation between perfusion pressure during CPB and postoperative neurologic defects. In recent studies by Feddersen et al.[114] and Arén et al.,[115] prostacyclin infusion was used to reduce platelet activation. Low arterial pressure (to 30 mm Hg or less), a side effect of prostacyclin, did not increase the incidence of postoperative cerebral dysfunction.

Several investigators have addressed the effect of lowered CPB pump flows with constant low pressures on the risk of cerebral injury during and after CPB. Studies by Ellis et al.[22] and by Kolkka and Hilberman[24] contended that the low flow/low pressure CPB technique utilized first by the Stanford group was not associated with increased postoperative neurologic or neuropsychologic complications.

CBF and factors influencing CBF in humans during CPB are less well documented and understood. In recent investigations by Henriksen et al.,[109] Govier et al.,[27] and Murkin et al.,[116] radioactive xenon 133 (^{133}Xe) was used to examine CBF during nonpulsatile CPB. In 1983 Henriksen et al.[109] measured CBF and addressed the relation between MAP and CBF in 29 patients during hypothermic CPB. They found that cerebral autoregulation was maintained down to arterial pressures as low as 55 mm Hg. When arterial pressures dropped below this level, there was a significant association between regional CBF and MAP during the hypothermic phase of CPB. This indicated an apparent loss of cerebral autoregulation. They also noted a 67 per cent increase in CBF during the hypothermic phase of CPB, reflecting "an uncoupling of flow and metabolism." They observed that "reactive hyperemia certainly indicates something is or was wrong." Cerebral emboli may produce an ischemic injury during an operation and permit hyperemia owing to the uncoupling of flow and metabolism.[117, 118]

In 1984 Govier et al.[27] studied the factors that influence regional CBF during nonpulsatile hypothermic CPB. Regional CBF was measured by radioactive ^{133}Xe clearance in 67 patients undergoing CABG. We found significant decreases in regional CBF (55 per cent) during CPB. Nasopharyngeal temperature and $PaCO_2$ were the only factors that significantly influenced CBF. Changes in regional CBF during CPB were directly related to changes in temperature and, presumably, to changes in cerebral metabolism. In our study there was a poor association between regional CBF and MAP. This finding is consistent with preserved autoregulation (Fig. 3–1).[27] In fact, during hypothermic CPB, the lower limit of autoregulation extended to MAPs as low as 30 mm Hg.

Murkin et al.[116] recently studied the influence of $PaCO_2$ on CBF during

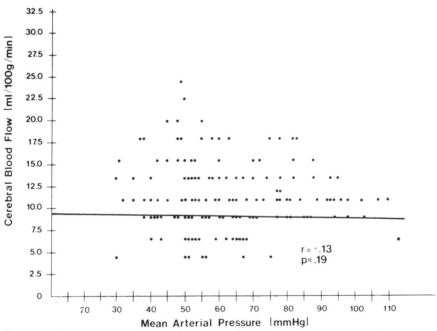

Figure 3–1. Cerebral blood flow versus mean arterial pressure during cardiopulmonary bypass. The line represents an average regression line over all patients. There are 44 hidden observations, that is, data points superimposed on one another.

hypothermic CPB. They demonstrated that the observations of Govier et al.[27] and Henriksen et al.[109] were not inconsistent. Differences in the acid–base management of each group accounted for much of the variation in CBF and cerebral autoregulation. We did not temperature-correct $Paco_2$[27]; thus the CBF measured reflected an actual $Paco_2$ that was significantly lower than that in the patients investigated by Henriksen's group (which used temperature-corrected $Paco_2$).[109] Murkin et al.[116] reported that a temperature-corrected $Paco_2$ of 40 mm Hg (pH-stat management) produced a profound cerebral hyperemia with significant uncoupling of oxygen supply and potential for damage during hypothermic CPB. This results in loss of cerebral autoregulation and may predispose patients to cerebral embolization because the elevated nonnutrient CBF is a greater fraction of total flow. When $Paco_2$ was not corrected for temperature (alpha-stat regimen), cerebral metabolic autoregulation remained intact and independent of MAP from 20 to 100 mm Hg.

There is disagreement over the optimal perfusion flow during hypothermic CPB. At times adequate surgical exposure may require very low perfusion flow rates. There is concern that CBF may be inadequate during these periods of low flow. Govier et al.[27] examined the effect of flow rates on regional CBF in ten patients by randomly varying flow and keeping other variables relatively constant. We found no significant change in regional CBF during hypothermic CPB when systemic blood flow was varied for short time intervals (minutes) between 1 and 2 L/min/m². This study suggests that with intact autoregulation, it may be possible to reduce perfusion flow rates during hypothermic bypass to as low as 1 L/min/m² for a short time without significantly reducing CBF and risking cerebral damage.

Some investigators believe that cerebrovascular occlusive disease, which is associated with increasing age, leads to inadequate cerebral perfusion.[5, 33, 103] It is unknown whether the pathophysiology of CBF in elderly patients is qualitatively different from that in younger patients. Structural alterations (e.g., cerebral atrophy) and cerebrovascular atherosclerosis appear to progressively reduce CBF with age.[119] Age, however, has not been shown to correlate with reduced CBF during CPB.[120]

In conclusion, rather than there being one single cause of the cerebral damage that follows CPB, there are many factors that may contribute to this damage.

CEREBRAL PROTECTION

Many therapies have been suggested to protect the brain against or lessen the severity of ischemic damage. The pathophysiology varies greatly among the different types of cerebral damage (global versus regional; anoxic versus hypoxic). Thus a particular therapy or drug cannot be expected to offer similar protection for all types of damage. Improving the balance between oxygen demand and supply is a major principle that underlies most current therapeutic management. What follows is a review of the therapies currently used to prevent and treat cerebral damage.

Inhibitors of Cerebral Metabolism

Hypothermia, which generally depresses metabolism, is currently by far the most effective and commonly used means of inhibiting cerebral metabolism during CPB.[121] The cerebral metabolic requirement for oxygen ($CMRO_2$) is reduced nonlinearly as temperature decreases. Hypothermia enhances the brain's tolerance of ischemia by slowing adenosine triphosphate depletion and lactic acid formation.[122] Hypothermia appears to depress general cerebral metabolism, whereas drugs, such as barbiturates, depress only that part related to active electrical function.[123] It is hypothermia's protective effect at the cellular level that seems to enable the brain to tolerate prolonged periods of circulatory arrest.[123–126]

Etomidate, a short-acting hypnotic, is also a potent depressant of $CMRO_2$. It is an anticonvulsant and reduces increased intracranial pressure. Etomidate appears to protect against various induced hypoxic-ischemic insults in animals.[127, 128]

Midazolam is a short-acting water-soluble benzodiazepine. In sufficient dosage it profoundly depresses $CMRO_2$ in dogs without severe hemodynamic depression or alteration of the cerebral energy state.[129] Accordingly, midazolam may be an alternative to barbiturates for cerebral protection.

It has been suggested that isoflurane, a volatile anesthetic, may be used to protect the brain during incomplete ischemia.[130] Isoflurane produces an isoelectric EEG in humans at hemodynamically tolerable concentrations (2.4 per cent).[131] It is believed that isoflurane protects the brain by decreasing $CMRO_2$, primarily by suppressing cortical electrical activity.[130, 131]

Barbiturates have been shown to protect the brain during incomplete ischemia.[124, 132–134] No consistent protection has been demonstrated during complete global ischemia.[135–138] Early animal studies demonstrated that barbiturates offer protection only if they are administered before, during, or shortly after the ischemic event.[134, 139–142] Barbiturates are known to reduce $CMRO_2$ in a dose-dependent manner but only down to the point of isoelectric EEG. Redution of $CMRO_2$ has been assumed to be the mechanism by which they protect the brain, but other possible mechanisms of protection have been suggested and are reviewed elsewhere.[105, 122, 143–145]

A prospective study by Slogoff et al.[26] of 204 mostly CABG patients undergoing normothermic CPB found that an improved neuropsychologic outcome was not achieved using 15 mg/kg of thiopental. In this 1982 study, patients undergoing intracardiac surgeries had a greater incidence of postoperative cerebral dysfunction than patients undergoing extracardiac operations. This study[26] led to a study by Nussmeier et al.[100] of 182 patients undergoing intracardiac procedures with normothermic CPB. They demonstrated that patients treated with thiopental (at an average dose of 39.5 mg/kg) starting before CPB and continuing throughout bypass had a significantly lower incidence of persistent neuropsychiatric complications (0 per cent) compared with those not given thiopental (7.5 per cent incidence). Nussmeier et al.[100] concluded that "barbiturate therapy did not appear to decrease the frequency of embolization, but rather did appear to reduce its clinical expression, presumably by decreasing the size of infarction." Although the large doses of thiopental resulted in a longer recovery time and an average 5-hour delay in extubation, these investigators recommend "the use of barbiturate therapy in patients undergoing intracardiac procedures to counteract the higher probability of postoperative neuropsychiatric complications in this population."[105] Unfortunately in this study CPB was normothermic and unfiltered.[146] It is therefore uncertain whether the results of this study can be directly applied to hypothermic filtered CPB. Not using in-line arterial filters possibly increased the incidence of embolization and subsequent neuropsychiatric complications.

Calcium Entry Blockers

There have been many studies of calcium's role in normal cellular function and during ischemia. In ischemia, extracellular calcium decreases—probably because it progressively enters the cells themselves.[147] This knowledge has led to many investigations of the potential of calcium entry blocking drugs to protect or minimize neurologic damage after ischemic events.[148–156] Nimodipine is one of the most extensively studied of the calcium entry blockers. Sakabe et al.[151] demonstrated (in a canine model) that nimodipine consistently prevented the delayed hypoperfusion state that otherwise occurs after ischemia. Nimodipine administered before complete cerebral ischemia improved the neurologic outcome in dogs and primates.[145, 149, 154] Sakabe et al.[151] reported that the calcium entry blocker nicardipine improves postischemic CBF. Nicardipine did not improve the neurologic outcome in dogs regardless of whether it was given before or after the ischemic period.

To date, the cerebral protective mechanism of calcium entry blockers, if it exists, is not known. Only a few human studies of these drugs have been completed, and they are not conclusive.[157–159] Therefore, whether calcium entry blockers actually protect the human brain during ischemia is unknown.

Antagonists of the Excitatory Amino Acid Receptors

A number of investigators are examining possible treatment of cerebral ischemia in animals by using pharmacologic agents that are antagonists at excitatory amino acid (EAA) receptors.[160-164] An enhanced release of EAA follows global cerebral ischemia.[160-162, 164] It has been postulated that these neurotransmitters contribute to the pathologic consequences of brain ischemia. Most of the investigators have found that these antagonists do indeed protect against focal and global ischemia in animals.[160-162, 164] Conversely, Block and Pulsinelli[163] showed that the EAA antagonist did not prevent ischemic neuronal damage in rats.

Other Cerebral Protective Agents

In animal models, phenytoin has been shown to provide cerebral protection after global cerebral ischemia.[165-167] Its mechanism of protection may be that it reduces the ion flux across membranes during cerebral hypoxia/anoxia and thereby decreases potassium accumulation.[165, 166]

Several animal studies indicate that lidocaine may protect the ischemic brain.[168-170] In pentobarbital-suppressed brains with flat EEGs (dogs), lidocaine delayed the efflux of potassium and further reduced metabolism by 15 per cent to 20 per cent.[169] Pretreatment with lidocaine significantly reduced the neural decrement and enhanced neural function recovery after acute cerebral ischemia induced by air embolism (cats).[170]

HYPERGLYCEMIA MANAGEMENT

Recent animal studies have shown that hyperglycemia greatly increased the severity of ischemic brain damage.[171, 172] In a retrospective study by Pulsinelli et al.,[173] the neurologic outcome of strokes in diabetics was significantly worse than that in nondiabetics. In addition, diabetics were more likely to suffer stroke-related deaths. In a separate prospective study of nondiabetic patients with ischemic strokes, Pulsinelli et al.[173] also showed that those with hyperglycemia had a poorer neurologic outcome. Berger and Hakim[174] had similar results in a retrospective review of 39 stroke patients. According to Sieber et al.,[175] "withholding glucose or giving it in moderation so as to keep the blood glucose below 200 mg/dL is recommended whenever brain ischemia may occur intraoperatively." This applies at any time during CPB.

Hyperbaric Oxygen Therapy

A number of authors have reported that hyperbaric oxygenation successfully treats massive air embolism that occurs during CPB.[176-178] The mechanisms of hyperbaric oxygen therapy include (a) reduction of the size of the gas emboli so that the area of distal ischemia resulting from the obstructed blood flow is reduced[179]; (b) dissolution of the large volume of oxygen in the plasma to facilitate oxygenation of ischemic tissue; and (c) reduction of the increased intracranial pressure caused by severe cerebral ischemia.[180]

CONCLUSION

Although there have been improvements in many aspects of CPB, ideal extracorporeal circulation is not yet available. Knowledge about the cause of the neurologic complications associated with CPB remains incomplete. Until more is known about the mechanisms of cerebral damage associated with CPB, their treatment or prevention cannot be firmly established. Given that this remains one of the most disturbing postoperative complications of cardiac surgery, we should continue to vigorously strive to understand and eliminate it.

References

1. Rimm AA: Trends in cardiac surgery in the United States. N Engl J Med 312:119–120, 1985.
2. Loop FD, Lytle BW, Gill CC, et al: Trends in selection and results of coronary artery reoperations. Ann Thorac Surg 36:380–388, 1983.
3. Reul GJ, Morris GC, Howell JF, et al: Current concepts in coronary artery surgery. Ann Thorac Surg 14:243–259, 1972.
4. Miller DC, Stinson EB, Oyer PE, et al: Discriminant analysis of the changing risks of coronary artery operations: 1971–1979. J Thorac Cardiovasc Surg 85:197–213, 1983.
5. Cosgrove DM, Loop FD, Lytle BW, et al: Primary myocardial revascularization. J Thorac Cardiovasc Surg 88:673–684, 1984.
6. Hutchinson JE, Green GE, Mekhjian HA, Kemp HG: Coronary bypass grafting in 376 consecutive patients, with three operative deaths. J Thorac Cardiovasc Surg 67:7–16, 1974.
7. Ashor GW, Meyer BW, Lindesmith GG, et al: Coronary artery disease. Arch Surg 107:30–33, 1973.
8. Gardner TJ, Horneffer PJ, Gott VL, et al: Coronary artery bypass grafting in women. Ann Surg 201:780–784, 1985.
9. Hall RJ, Elayda MA, Gray A, et al: Coronary artery bypass: Long-term follow up of 22,284 consecutive patients. Circulation 68(suppl 2):20–26, 1983.
10. Kouchoukos NT, Oberman A, Kirklin JW, et al: Coronary bypass surgery: Analysis of factors affecting hospital mortality. Circulation 62(suppl 1):84–89, 1980.
11. Loop FD, Cosgrove DM, Lytle BW, et al: An 11 year evolution of coronary arterial surgery (1967–1978). Ann Surg 190:444–455, 1979.

12. Ehrenhaft JL, Claman MA, Layton JM, Zimmerman GR: Cerebral complications of open heart surgery: Further observations. J Thorac Cardiovasc Surg 42:514–526, 1961.
13. Gilman S: Cerebral disorders after open heart operations. N Engl J Med 272:439–498, 1965.
14. Kornfeld DS, Zimberg S, Malm JR: Psychiatric complications of open heart surgery. N Engl J Med 273:287–292, 1965.
15. Gilberstadt H, Sako Y: Intellectual and personality changes following open heart surgery. Arch Gen Psychiatry 16:210–214, 1967.
16. Tufo HM, Ostfeld AM, Shekelle R: Central nervous system dysfunction following open heart surgery. JAMA 212:1333–1340, 1970.
17. Lee WH, Brady MP, Rowe JM, Miller WC Jr: Effects of extracorporeal circulation upon behavior, personality, and brain function. Part 2. Hemodynamic metabolic, and psychometric correlations. Ann Surg 173:1013–1023, 1971.
18. Branthwaite MA: Neurological damage related to open heart surgery: A clinical survey. Thorax 27:748–753, 1972.
19. Stockard JJ, Bickford RG, Schauble JF: Pressure-dependent cerebral ischemia during cardiopulmonary bypass. Neurology 23:521, 1973.
20. Branthwaite MA: Prevention of neurological damage during open heart surgery. Thorax 30:258–260, 1975.
21. Åberg T, Kihlgren M: Cerebral protection during open heart surgery. Thorax 32:525–533, 1977.
22. Ellis RJ, Wisniewski A, Potts R, et al: Reduction of flow rate and arterial pressure at moderate hypothermia does not result in cerebral dysfunction. J Thorac Cardiovasc Surg 79:173–180, 1980.
23. Breuer AC, Furlan AJ, Hanson MR, et al: Neurologic complications of open heart surgery: Computer associated analysis of 531 patients. Cleve Clin Q 48:205–206, 1981.
24. Kolkka R, Hilberman M: Neurologic dysfunction following cardiac operation with low-flow, low-pressure cardiopulmonary bypass. J Thorac Cardiovasc Surg 79:432–437, 1980.
25. Turnipseed WD, Berkoff HA, Belzer FO: Postoperative stroke in cardiac and peripheral vascular disease. Ann Surg 192:365–368, 1980.
26. Slogoff ST, Girgis KZ, Keats AS: Etiologic factors in neuropsychiatric complications associated with cardiopulmonary bypass. Anesth Analg 61:903–911, 1982.
27. Govier AV, Reves JG, McKay RD, et al: Factors and their influence on regional cerebral blood flow during nonpulsatile cardiopulmonary bypass. Ann Thorac Surg 38:592–600, 1984.
28. Sotaniemi KA: Cerebral outcome after extracorporeal circulation: Comparison between prospective and retrospective evaluations. Arch Neurol 40:75–77, 1983.
29. Bjork VO, Hultquist G: Brain damage in children after deep hypothermia for open heart surgery. Thorax 15:284–291, 1960.
30. Brierley JB: Neuropathological findings in patients dying after open heart surgery. Thorax 18:291–304, 1963.
31. Aguilar MJ, Gerbode F, Hill JD: Neuropathologic complications of cardiac surgery. J Thorac Cardiovasc Surg 61:676–685, 1971.
32. Sotaniemi KA: Brain damage and neurological outcome after open heart surgery. J Neurol Neurosurg Psychiatry 43:127–135, 1980.
33. Shaw PJ, Bates D, Cartlidge NEF, et al: Early neurological complications of coronary artery bypass surgery. Br Med J 291:1384–1387, 1985.
34. Shaw PJ: Neurological complications of cardiovascular surgery: Procedures involving the heart and thoracic aorta. CNS sequelae of heart surgery. Anesthesiol Clin 24:159–200, 1986.
35. Hill JD, Aguilar MJ, Baranco A, et al: Neuropathological manifestations of cardiac surgery. Ann Thorac Surg 7:409–419, 1969.
36. Heller SS, Frank KA, Malm JR, et al: Psychiatric complications of open heart surgery. N Engl J Med 28:1015–1020, 1970.
37. Javid H, Tufo HM, Najafi H, et al: Neurological abnormalities following open heart surgery. J Thorac Cardiovasc Surg 58:502–509, 1969.

38. Hansotia PL, Myers WO, Ray JF III, et al: Prognostic value of electroencephalography in cardiac surgery. Ann Thoracic Surg 19:127–134, 1975.
39. Cannom DS, Miller DC, Shumway NE, et al: The long-term followup of patients undergoing saphenous vein bypass surgery. Circulation 49:77–85, 1974.
40. Branthwaite MA: Detection of neurological damage during open heart surgery. Thorax 28:464–472, 1973.
41. Hodgman JR, Cosgrove DM: Post-hospital course and complications following coronary bypass surgery. Cleve Clin Q 43:125–129, 1976.
42. Lee MC, Geiger J, Nicoloff D, Klasse AC: Cerebrovascular complications associated with coronary artery bypass (CAB) procedure. Fourth Joint Meeting on Stroke and Cerebral Circulation, Vienna, Austria, p. 107, 1979.
43. Gonzalez-Scarano F, Hurtig HL: Neurologic complications of coronary artery bypass grafting: Case-control study. Neurology 31:1032–1035, 1981.
44. Muraoka R, Yokota M, Aoshima M, et al: Subclinical changes in brain morphology following cardiac operations as reflected by computed tomographic scans of the brain. J Thorac Cardiovasc Surg 81:364–369, 1981.
45. Breuer AC, Furlan AJ, Hanson MR: Central nervous system complications of coronary artery bypass graft surgery: Prospective analysis of 421 patients. Stroke 14:682–687, 1983.
46. Heikkinen L, Harjula A, Mattila S: Neurological events in cardiac surgery. Ann Chir Gynaecol 74:118–123, 1985.
47. Furlan AJ, Breuer AC: Central nervous system complications of open heart surgery. Stroke 15:912–915, 1984.
48. Breuer AC, Furlan AJ, Hanson MR, et al: Comparative risk of stroke during left heart valve surgery versus coronary artery bypass: Mechanism of stroke in open heart surgery. Neurology 31:107, 1981.
49. Gardner TJ, Horneffer PJ, Manolio TA, et al: Stroke following coronary artery bypass grafting: A ten year study. Ann Thorac Surg 40:575–581, 1985.
50. Gersh BJ, Kronmal RA, Frye RL: Coronary arteriography and coronary artery bypass surgery: Morbidity and mortality in patients age 65 years or older. Circulation 67:483–491, 1983.
51. Hibler BA, Wright JO, Wright CB, et al: Coronary artery bypass surgery in the elderly. Arch Surg 118:402–404, 1983.
52. Faro RS, Golden MD, Javid H, et al: Coronary revascularization in septuagenarians. J Thorac Cardiovasc Surg 86:616–620, 1983.
53. Knapp WS, Douglas JS, Craver JM, et al: Efficacy of coronary artery bypass grafting in elderly patients with coronary artery disease. Am J Cardiol 47:923–930, 1981.
54. Breuer AC, Franco I, Marzewski D, Soto-Velasco J: Left ventricular thrombi seen by ventriculography are a significant risk factor for stroke in open heart surgery. Ann Neurol 10:103–104, 1981.
55. Barnes RW, Liebman PR, Marszalek PB, et al: The natural history of asymptomatic carotid disease in patients undergoing cardiovascular surgery. Surgery 90:1075–1083, 1981.
56. Jones EL, Craver JM, Michalik RA, et al: Combined carotid and coronary operations: When are they necessary? J Thorac Cardiovasc Surg 87:7–16, 1984.
57. Ivey TD, Strandness DE, Williams DB: Management of patients with carotid bruit undergoing cardiopulmonary bypass. J Thorac Cardiovasc Surg 87:183–189, 1984.
58. Edgerton N, Kay JH: Psychological disturbances associated with open heart surgery. Br J Psychiatry 110:433–439, 1964.
59. Blanchy PH, Starr A: Post-cardiotomy delirium. Am J Psychiatry 86:371–375, 1964.
60. Cohen SI: Neurological and psychiatric aspects of open heart surgery. Thorax 19:575–578, 1964.
61. Rabiner CJ, Willner AE: Psychopathology observed on follow up after coronary bypass surgery. J Nerv Ment Dis 162:295–301, 1976.
62. Blanchy PH, Kloster FE: Relation of cardiac output to post-cardiotomy delirium. J Thorac Cardiovasc Surg 53:422–427, 1966.
63. Calabrese JR, Skwerer RG, Gulledge AD, et al: Incidence of postoperative delirium following myocardial revascularization. Cleve Clin J Med 54:29–32, 1987.

64. Kornfeld DS, Heller SS, Frank KA, et al: Delirium after coronary artery bypass surgery. J Thorac Cardiovasc Surg 76:93–96, 1978.
65. Savageau JA, Stanton BA, Jenkins CD, Klein MD: Neuropsychological dysfunction following elective cardiac operation. J Thorac Cardiovasc Surg 84:585–594, 1982.
66. Gotze P, Huse-Kleinstoll G, Speidel H: Psychic and neurological dysfunctions after open-heart-surgery: A review of the present state of research. In Speidel H, Rodewald G (eds): Psychic and Neurological Dysfunctions After Open-Heart Surgery. New York, Thieme Stratton, 1980, pp 6–13.
67. Barash P: Cardiopulmonary bypass and postoperative neurologic dysfunction. Am Heart J 99:675–677, 1980.
68. Sotaniemi KA, Juolasmaa AN, Hokkanen ET: Neuropsychologic outcome after open heart surgery. Arch Neurol 38:2–8, 1981.
69. Smith PL, Newman SP, Ell PJ, et al: Cerebral consequences of cardiopulmonary bypass. Lancet 1:823–825, 1986.
70. Sotaniemi KA, Mononen H, Hokkanen TE: Long term cerebral outcome after open heart surgery. Stroke 17:410–416, 1986.
71. Dubin WR, Field HL, Gastfriend DR: Postcardiotomy delirium: A critical review. J Thorac Cardiovasc Surg 77:586–594, 1979.
72. Pedley TA, Emerson RG: Neurological complications of cardiac surgery. In Matthews LJ, Glaser RG (eds): Recent Advances in Clinical Neurology. Edinburgh, Churchill Livingstone, 1984.
73. Savageau JA, Stanton BA, Jenkins CD, Frater RWM: Neuropsychological dysfunction following elective cardiac operation. J Thorac Cardiovasc Surg 84:595–600, 1982.
74. Mayou R: Invited review: The psychiatric and social consequences of coronary artery surgery. J Psychosom Res 30:255–271, 1986.
75. Shaw PJ, Bates D, Cartlidge NEF, et al: Early intellectual dysfunction following coronary bypass surgery. Q J Med 58:59–68, 1986.
76. Priest WS, Zaks MS, Yacorzynski GK, Boshes B: The neurologic, psychiatric and psychologic aspects of cardiac surgery. Med Clin North Am 41:155–169, 1957.
77. Åberg T, Tyden H, Ronquist G, et al: Release of adenylate kinase into cerebrospinal fluid during open heart surgery and its relation to postoperative intellectual function. Lancet 1:1139–1142, 1982.
78. Frank KA, Heller SS, Kornfeld DS, Malm JR: Long-term effects of open heart surgery on intellectual functioning. J Thorac Cardiovasc Surg 64:811–815, 1972.
79. Juolasmaa A, Outakoski J, Hirvenoja R, et al: Effect of open heart surgery on intellectual performance. J Clin Neurol 3:181–197, 1981.
80. Åberg T: Effect of open heart surgery on intellectual function. Scand J Thorac Cardiovasc Surg [Suppl] 15:3–63, 1974.
81. Raymond M, Conklin C, Schaeffer J, et al: Coping with transient intellectual dysfunction after coronary bypass surgery. Heart Lung 13:531–539, 1984.
82. Åberg T, Ronquist G, Tyden H, et al: Adverse effects in the brain in cardiac operations as assessed by biochemical, psychometric and radiologic methods. J Thorac Cardiovasc Surg 87:99–105, 1984.
83. Patterson RH, Wasser JS, Porro RS: The effect of various filters on microembolic cerebrovascular blockade following cardiopulmonary bypass. Ann Thorac Surg 17:464–473, 1974.
84. Loop FD, Szabo J, Rowlinson RD, Urbanek K: Events related to microembolism during extracorporeal perfusion in man: Effectiveness of in-line filtration recorded by ultrasound. Ann Thorac Surg 21:412–420, 1976.
85. Sachdev NS, Carter CC, Swank RL, Blachly PH: Relationship between postcardiotomy delirium, clinical neurological changes and EEG abnormalities. J Thorac Cardiovasc Surg 54:557–563, 1967.
86. Allardyce DB, Yoshida SH, Ashmore PG: The importance of microembolism in the pathogenesis of organ dysfunction caused by prolonged use of the pump oxygenator. Microembolism 52:706–715, 1966.
87. Oka Y, Moriwaki KM, Hong Y, et al: Detection of air emboli in the left heart by M-mode transesophageal echocardiography following cardiopulmonary bypass. Anesthesiology 63:109–113, 1985.

88. Fish KJ: Microembolization: Etiology and prevention. In Hilberman M (ed): Brain Injury and Protection During Heart Surgery. Boston, Martinus Nijhoff, 1987, pp 67–83.
89. Swank RL: Alteration of blood on storage: Measurement of adhesiveness of "aging" platelets and leukocytes and their removal by filtration. N Engl J Med 265:728–733, 1961.
90. Thomassen RW, Howbert JP, Winn DF, Thompson SW: The occurrence and characterization of emboli associated with the use of a silicone antifoaming agent. J Thorac Cardiovasc Surg 41:611–622, 1961.
91. Cassie AB, Riddell AG, Yates PO: Hazard of antifoam emboli from a bubble oxygenator. Thorax 15:22–29, 1960.
92. Allen P: Central nervous system emboli in open heart surgery. Can J Surg 6:332–337, 1963.
93. Nicks R: Arterial air embolism. Thorax 22:320–326, 1967.
94. Solis RT, Noon GP, Beall AC, DeBakey ME: Particulate microembolism during cardiac operation. Ann Thorac Surg 17:332–344, 1974.
95. Taylor KM: Brain damage during open heart surgery. Thorax 37:873–876, 1982.
96. Spencer FC, Rossi NP, Yu S, Koepke JA: The significance of air embolism during cardiopulmonary bypass. J Thorac Cardiovasc Surg 19:615–634, 1965.
97. Rodigas PC, Meyer FJ, Haasler GB, et al: Intraoperative 2-dimensional echocardiography: Ejection of microbubbles from the left ventricle after cardiac surgery. Am J Cardiol 50:1130–1132, 1982.
98. Aris A, Solanes H, Camara ML, et al: Arterial line filtration during cardiopulmonary bypass. J Thorac Cardiovasc Surg 91:526–533, 1986.
99. Ehrenhaft JL, Claman MA, Layton JM, Zimmerman GR: Cerebral complications of open-heart surgery: Further observations. J Thorac Cardiovasc Surg 42:514–526, 1961.
100. Nussmeier NA, Arlund C, Slogoff S: Neuropsychiatric complications after cardiopulmonary bypass: Cerebral protection by a barbiturate. Anesthesiology 64:165–170, 1986.
101. Martin WRW, Hashimoto SA: Stroke in coronary bypass surgery. Can Sciences Neurol 9:21–26, 1982.
102. Dobkin BH: Emboli and open heart surgery. Neurology 33:1247, 1983.
103. Parker FB, Marvasti MA, Bove EL: Neurologic complications following coronary artery bypass. The role of atherosclerotic emboli. J Thorac Cardiovasc Surg 33:207–209, 1985.
104. Mills NL, Ochsner JL: Massive air embolism during cardiopulmonary bypass: Causes, prevention and management. J Thorac Cardiovasc Surg 80:708–717, 1980.
105. Nussmeier NA, McDermott JP: Macroembolization: Prevention and outcome modification. In Hilberman (ed): Brain Injury and Protection During Heart Surgery. Boston, Martinus Nijhoff, 1987, pp 85–107.
106. Silverstien A, Krieger HP: Neurologic complications of cardiac surgery. Arch Neurol 5:135–139, 1960.
107. Bounds JV, Sandok BA, Barnhorst DA: Fatal cerebral embolism following aortocoronary bypass graft surgery. Stroke 7:611–614, 1976.
108. McKibbin DW, Bulkley BH, Green WR, et al: Fatal cerebral atheromatous embolization after cardiopulmonary bypass. J Thorac Cardiovasc Surg 71:741–745, 1976.
109. Henriksen L, Hjelms E, Lindeburgh T: Brain hyperperfusion during cardiac operations. J Thorac Cardiovasc Surg 86:202–208, 1983.
110. Bojar RM, Najafi H, DeLaria GA, et al: Neurological complications of coronary revascularization. Ann Thorac Surg 36:427–432, 1983.
111. Henriksen L: Evidence suggestive of diffuse brain damage following cardiac operations. Lancet 2:816–820, 1984.
112. Stockard JJ, Bickford RG, Myers RR, et al: Hypotension-induced changes in cerebral function during cardiac surgery. Stroke 5:730–746, 1974.
113. Heikkinen L: Clinically significant neurological disorders following open heart surgery. J Thorac Cardiovasc Surg 33:201–206, 1985.
114. Feddersen K, Arén C, Nilsson NJ, Radegran K: Cerebral blood flow and metabolism

during cardiopulmonary bypass with special reference to effects of hypotension induced by prostacyclin. Ann Thorac Surg 41:395–400, 1986.

115. Arén C, Blomstrand C, Wikkelso C, Radegran K: Hypotension induced by prostacyclin treatment during cardiopulmonary bypass does not increase the risk of cerebral complications. J Thorac Cardiovasc Surg 88:748–753, 1984.

116. Murkin JM, Farrar JK, Tweed WA, et al: Cerebral autoregulation and flow/metabolism coupling during cardiopulmonary bypass: The influence of $Paco_2$. Anesth Analg 66:825–832, 1987.

117. Lenzi GL, Frackowiak RSJ, Jones T: Cerebral oxygen metabolism and blood flow in human cerebral ischemic infarction. J Cereb Blood Flow Metab 2:321–335, 1982.

118. Lassen NA: The luxury-perfusion syndrome and its possible relation to acute metabolic acidosis localized within the brain. Lancet 2:113, 1966.

119. Naritomi H, Meyer JS, Sakai F, et al: Effects of advancing age on regional cerebral blood flow. Arch Neurol 36:410–416, 1979.

120. Brusino FG, Reves JG, Prough DS, et al: The effect of age on cerebral blood flow autoregulation during hypothermic cardiopulmonary bypass. Anesthesiology 67:A10, 1987.

121. Gisvold SE, Steen PA: Drug therapy in brain ischaemia. Br J Anaesth 57:96–109, 1985.

122. Safar P, Bleyaert A, Nemoto EM, et al: Resuscitation after global brain ischemia–anoxia. Crit Care Med 6:215–227, 1978.

123. Michenfelder JD: The interdependency of cerebral functional and metabolic effects following massive doses of thiopental in the dog. Anesthesiology 41:231–236, 1974.

124. Michenfelder JD, Milde JH, Sundt TM: Cerebral protection by barbiturate anesthesia. Arch Neurol 33:345–350, 1976.

125. Carlsson C, Hagerdal M, Siesjo BK: Protective effect of hypothermia in cerebral oxygen deficiency caused by arterial hypoxia. Anesthesiology 44:27–35, 1976.

126. Siebke H, Rod T, Breivik H, Lind B: Survival after 40 minutes' submersion without cerebral sequelae. Lancet 1:1275–1277, 1975.

127. Van Reempts J, Borgers M, Van Eyndhoven J, Hermans C: Protective effects of etomidate in hypoxic-ischemic brain damage in the rat. A morphologic assessment. Exp Neurol 76:181–195, 1982.

128. Wauquier A: Profile of etomidate. Anaesthesia 38(suppl):26–33, 1983.

129. Nugent M, Artru AA, Michenfelder JD: Cerebral metabolic, vascular and protective effects of midazolam maleate. Anesthesiology 56:172–176, 1982.

130. Newberg LA, Michenfelder JD: Cerebral protection by isoflurane during hypoxemia or ischemia. Anesthesiology 59:29–35, 1983.

131. Newberg LA, Milde JH, Michenfelder JD: The cerebral metabolic effects of isoflurane at and above concentrations that suppress cortical electrical activity. Anesthesiology 59:23–28, 1983.

132. Smith AL, Hoff JT, Nielsen SL, Larson CP: Barbiturate protection in acute focal cerebral ischemia. Stroke 5:1–7, 1974.

133. Selman WR, Spetzler RF, Roessmann UR: Barbiturate-induced coma therapy for focal cerebral ischemia. J Neurosurg 55:220–226, 1981.

134. Hoff JT, Marshall L: Barbiturates in neurosurgery. Clin Neurosurg 26:637–642, 1979.

135. Michenfelder JD: Cerebral preservation for intraoperative focal ischemia. Clin Neurosurg 32:105–113, 1985.

136. Steen PA, Milde JH, Michenfelder JD: No barbiturate protection in a dog model of complete cerebral ischema. Ann Neurol 5:343–340, 1979.

137. Gisvold SE, Safar P, Hendricks HHL, et al: Thiopental treatment after global brain ischemia in pigtailed monkeys. Anesthesiology 60:88–96, 1984.

138. Abramson NS, Safar P, Detre K, et al: Results of a randomized clinical trial of brain resuscitation with thiopental. Anesthesiology 59:A101, 1983.

139. Bleyaert AL, Nemoto EM, Safar P, et al: Thiopental amelioration of brain damage after global ischemia in monkeys. Anesthesiology 49:390–398, 1978.

140. Corkill G, Chikovani OK, McLeish I, et al: Timing of pentobarbital administration for brain protection in experimental stroke. Surg Neurol 5:147–149, 1976.

141. Corkill G, Sivalingam S, Reitan JA, et al: Dose dependency of the post-insult protective effect of pentobarbital in the canine experimental stroke model. Stroke 9:10–12, 1978.

142. Meyer FB, Sundt TM, Yanagihara T, Anderson RE: Focal cerebral ischemia: Patho-physiologic mechanisms and rationale for future avenues of treatment. Mayo Clin Proc 62:35–55, 1987.
143. Shapiro HM: Barbiturates in brain ischaemia. Br J Anaesth 57:82–95, 1985.
144. Kirsch JR, Dean JM, Rogers MC: Current concepts in brain resuscitation. Arch Intern Med 146:1413–1419, 1986.
145. Steen PA, Michenfelder JD: Cerebral protection with barbiturates: A relation to anesthetic effect. Stroke 9:140–142, 1978.
146. Nussmeier N: Personal communication, 1988.
147. Harris RJ, Symon L, Branston NM, Bayhan M: Changes in extracellular calcium activity in cerebral ischaemia. J Cereb Blood Flow Metab 1:203–209, 1981.
148. Deshpande JK, Wieloch T: Flunarizine, a calcium entry blocker, ameliorates ischemic brain damage in the rat. Anesthesiology 64:215–224, 1986.
149. Steen PA, Newberg LA, Milde JH, Michenfelder JD: Nimodipine improves cerebral blood flow and neurologic recovery after complete cerebral ischemia in the dog. J Cereb Blood Flow Metab 3:38–43, 1983.
150. Young WL, Josovitz K, Morales O, Chien S: The effect of nimodipine on postischemic cerebral glucose utilization and blood flow in the rat. Anesthesiology 67:54–59, 1987.
151. Sakabe T, Nagai I, Ishikawa T, et al: Nicardipine increased post-ischemic cerebral blood flow without improving neurological outcome. J Cereb Blood Flow Metab 6:684–690, 1986.
152. Harris RJ, Branston NM, Symon L, et al: The effects of a calcium antagonist, nimodipine, upon physiological responses of cerebral vasculature and its possible influence upon focal cerebral ischaemia. Stroke 13:759–766, 1982.
153. Mohamed AA, Gotoh O, Graham DI, et al: Effect of pretreatment with the calcium antagonist nimodipine on local cerebral blood flow and histopathology after middle cerebral artery occlusion. Ann Neurol 18:705–711, 1985.
154. Steen PA, Newberg LA, Milde JH, Michenfelder JD: Cerebral blood flow and neurologic outcome when nimodipine is given after complete cerebral ischemia in the dog. J Cereb Blood Flow Metab 4:82–87, 1984.
155. Mohamed AA, McCulloch J, Mendelow AD, et al: Effect of the calcium antagonist nimodipine on local cerebral blood flow: Relationship to arterial blood pressure. J Cereb Blood Flow Metab 4:206–211, 1984.
156. Steen PA, Gisvold SE, Milde JH, et al: Nimodipine improves outcome when given after complete cerebral ischemia in primates. Anesthesiology 64:406–414, 1985.
157. Allen GS, Ahn HS, Preziosi TJ, et al: Cerebral arterial spasms—a controlled trial of nimodipine in patients with subarachnoid hemorrhage. N Engl J Med 308:619–624, 1983.
158. Gelmers HJ: The effects of nimodipine on the clinical course of patients with acute ischemic stroke. Acta Neurol Scand 69:232–239, 1984.
159. Gelmers HJ: Calcium-channel blockers: Effects on cerebral blood flow and potential uses for acute stroke: Am J Cardiol 55:144B–148B, 1985.
160. Duverger D, Benavides J, Cudennec A, et al: A glutamate antagonist reduces infarction size following focal cerebral ischaemia independently of vascular and metabolic changes. J Cereb Blood Flow Metab 7(suppl 1):S144, 1987.
161. Swan JH, Evans MC, Meldrum BS: Ischaemic brain damage: Protection by 2-chloroad-enosine, a modulator of excitatory neurotransmission. J Cereb Blood Flow Metab 7(suppl 1):X145, 1987.
162. Oyzurt E, Graham DI, McCulloch J, et al: The NMDA receptor antagonist MK-801 reduces focal ischaemic brain damage in the cat. J Cereb Blood Flow Metab 7(suppl 1):S146, 1987.
163. Block GA, Pulsinelli WA: Excitatory amino acid receptor antagonists: Failure to prevent ischemic neuronal damage. J Cereb Blood Flow Metab 7(suppl 1):S149, 1987.
164. Gill R, Foster AC, Iversen IL, et al: Ischaemia-induced degeneration of hippocampal neurones in gerbils is prevented by systemic administration of MK-801. J Cereb Blood Flow Metab 7(suppl 1):S153, 1987.

165. Artru AA, Michenfelder JD: Cerebral protective, metabolic, and vascular effects of phenytoin. Stroke 11:377–382, 1980.
166. Artru AA, Michenfelder JD: Anoxic cerebral potassium accumulation reduced by phenytoin: Mechanism of cerebral protection? Anesth Analg 60:41–45, 1981.
167. Cullen JP, Aldrete JA, Jankovsky L, Romo-Salas F: Protective action of phenytoin in cerebral ischemia. Anesth Analg 58:165–169, 1979.
168. Astrup J, Sørensen PM, Sørensen HR: Inhibition of cerebral oxygen and glucose consumption in the dog by hypothermia, pentobarbital and lidocaine. Anesthesiology 55:263–268, 1981.
169. Astrup J, Skøvsted P, Gjerris F, Sørensen HR: Increase in extracellular potassium in the brain during circulatory arrest: Effects of hypothermia, lidocaine, and thiopental. Anesthesiology 55:256–262, 1981.
170. Evans DE, Kobrine AI, LeGrys DC, Bradley ME: Protective effect of lidocaine in acute cerebral ischemia induced by air embolism. J Neurosurg 60:257–263, 1984.
171. Ginsberg MD, Welsh FA, Budd WW: Deleterious effect of glucose pretreatment on recovery from diffuse cerebral ischemia in the cat. Stroke 11:347–354, 1980.
172. Pulsinelli WA, Levy DE, Duffy TE: Regional cerebral blood flow and glucose metabolism following transient forebrain ischemia. Ann Neurology 11:499–509, 1982.
173. Pulsinelli WA, Levy DE, Sigsbee B, et al: Increased damage after ischemic stroke in patients with hyperglycemia with or without established diabetes mellitus. Am J Med 74:540–544, 1983.
174. Berger L, Hakim AM: The association of hyperglycemia with cerebral edema in stroke. Stroke 17:865–897, 1986.
175. Sieber FE, Smith DS, Traystman RJ, Wollman H: Glucose: A reevaluation of its intraoperative use. Anesthesiology 67:72–81, 1987.
176. Steward D, Williams WG, Freedom R: Hypothermia in conjunction with hyperbaric oxygenation in the treatment of massive air embolism during cardiopulmonary bypass. Ann Thor Surg 24:591–593, 1977.
177. Takita H, Oiszewski W, Schimert G, Lanphier EH: Hyperbaric treatment of cerebral air embolism as a result of open-heart surgery. Report of a case. J Thorac Cardiovasc Surg 55:682–685, 1968.
178. Toscano M, Chiavarelli R, Ruvolo G, et al: Management of massive air embolism during open-heart surgery with retrograde perfusion of the cerebral vessels and hyperbaric oxygenation. J Thorac Cardiovasc Surg 31:183–184, 1983.
179. Myers RA, Schnitzer BM: Hyperbaric oxygen use. Update 1984. Postgrad Med 76:83–95, 1984.
180. Murphy BP, Harford FJ, Cramer FS: Cerebral air embolism resulting from invasive medical procedures. Treatment with hyperbaric oxygen. Ann Surg 201:242–245, 1985.

ANESTHESIA DURING CARDIOPULMONARY BYPASS: Does It Matter?

J. G. REVES, NARDA CROUGHWELL, JAMES R. JACOBS, and WILLIAM GREELEY

In the United States during 1986, 480,000 patients were anesthetized for cardiac surgical procedures that involved use of cardiopulmonary bypass (CPB). Despite this large clinical experience, little is known about anesthesia and CPB. This chapter explores our knowledge concerning two questions about anesthesia and CPB: (1) Does CPB change the kinetics of anesthetic drugs given during bypass? (2) Does anesthesia affect the patient's response to CPB?

KINETICS OF ANESTHETIC DRUGS DURING CARDIOPULMONARY BYPASS

The effects of CPB on the pharmacokinetics of drugs have been reviewed previously.[1, 2] Intravenous drugs can be given into the peripheral or central venous circulations, into the pump oxygenator venous reservoir, or into the arterial inflow line (though the danger of air embolus is considerable with the latter route). The most reliable route is into the venous reservoir.[3] Uptake and elimination of inhalation anesthetics are also effective by means of the pump oxygenator.[4] It is postulated that the physiologic and physical aspects (e.g., hypotension, hemodilution, redistribution of blood flow, hypothermia, lung isolation, and the membrane oxygenator) of CPB may be pharmacokinetically relevant to alterations in drug disposition. Theoretically, all major pharmacokinetic processes should be affected by CPB.

Many of the studies in which drug blood levels during or after CPB have been analyzed are summarized in Table 4–1. This qualitative

TABLE 4–1. STUDIES OF PHARMACOKINETICS AND CARDIOPULMONARY BYPASS

Drug	Summary of Authors' Findings	Reference
Alfentanil	The free alfentanil concentration did not decline markedly at the start of CPB, although the total alfentanil concentration fell by half. After CPB, the elimination half-life was more than double that pre-CPB and was related to a similar increase in the distribution volume, with no change in alfentanil clearance. Free fraction was markedly higher after CPB than before CPB.	5
Alfentanil and fentanyl	In vitro experiments showed that fentanyl, but not alfentanil, was sequestered by the extracorporeal circuit. The absorption of fentanyl was pH dependent and time related.	65
Alfentanil and fentanyl	During continuous infusions of alfentanil or fentanyl, commencement of CPB was associated with decreases in plasma opiate concentrations.	50
Alphaxalone	During continuous infusion of alphaxalone, drug plasma concentrations fell with the commencement of CPB, tended to rise during the period of active cooling, and then remained relatively stable until the time of rewarming, at which point the levels generally fell slightly. The final concentrations of alphaxalone showed no relation to either length of CPB or duration of hypothermia and were comparable to levels reported in patients undergoing other types of surgery, suggesting the CPB had little effect on the plasma concentrations of alphaxalone at the end of surgery.	64
Cefamandole	Compared with that in patients not undergoing surgery, elimination of cefamandole was prolonged during CPB.	66
Cefazolin	After intramuscular administration of cefazolin at the time of premedication, plasma cefazolin levels fell at the start of CPB and remained stable for the duration of CPB.	67
Cefazolin	Serum cefazolin levels dropped abruptly on initiation of CPB and the duration of CPB. The elimination half-life was markedly increased during CPB, but no additional decrease in the renal excretion of cefazolin beyond that caused by anesthesia and thoracotomy was noted. The volume of distribution increased significantly during surgery and CPB.	68
Cephalothin	Cephalothin concentrations dropped on initiation of CPB and were relatively constant thereafter. Surgery and CPB had little effect on renal clearance of cephalothin, but they decreased metabolic clearance of the drug, resulting in a prolonged elimination half-life.	69
Digitoxin	Digitoxin levels fell on initiation of CPB and then rebounded to preoperative levels by the first postoperative day, in parallel with changes in hematocrit.	70
Digoxin	In a series of studies abstracted by Holley et al., digoxin levels were found to fall with the initiation of CPB and then tended to rise after termination of CPB, depending on the degree to which renal function was impaired by CPB.	1

TABLE 4–1. STUDIES OF PHARMACOKINETICS AND CARDIOPULMONARY BYPASS *Continued*

Drug	Summary of Authors' Findings	Reference
d-Tubocurarine	During continuous infusion of d-tubocurarine (dTc), there was either an immediate or a gradual rise in the plasma dTc concentrations on institution of CPB, which was followed by a plateau. After CPB (and termination of the infusion), plasma dTc concentrations fell at a rate slower than in normal patients, both renal and total plasma clearance being impaired. The free concentration of dTc changed roughly in parallel and in proportion to the changes in total dTc levels.	71
Enflurane, isoflurane, and halothane	In an in vitro model consisting of a roller pump and bubble oxygenator primed with whole blood and crystalloid, data were obtained suggesting that uptake of isoflurane and enflurane administered through a bubble oxygenator and elimination of isoflurane are more rapid than for halothane, as was expected because of the lower blood solubility of isoflurane and enflurane. Increasing pump flow had no significant effect, but increasing the rate of gas inflow did.	4
Fentanyl	After an infusion of fentanyl that ended well before CPB, fentanyl levels fell with the initiation of CPB but then remained relatively constant for the remainder of CPB and for the first hour after discontinuation of CPB.	72
Fentanyl	After a bolus of fentanyl for induction and maintenance of anesthesia, plasma fentanyl concentrations fell by about 50 per cent with the initiation of CPB and remained relatively unchanged until 2 hours post CPB, whereupon they fell with a prolonged elimination of half-life.	73
Fentanyl	After bolus administration of fentanyl before CPB, plasma fentanyl levels dropped profoundly on initiating bypass and then remained relatively constant until the end of CPB, whereupon they increased and then declined with an elimination half-life that was prolonged in comparison to surgical controls. The increased half-life correlated with a decrease in hepatic perfusion, both during and after CPB.	74
Fentanyl	After a bolus of fentanyl at induction of anesthesia, plasma fentanyl concentrations, total protein, albumin, and hematocrit declined with initiation of CPB but remained unchanged thereafter. Pulmonary artery fentanyl concentrations were higher than systemic arterial concentrations during bypass, but when lung ventilation and perfusion were restored, radial artery concentrations rose above concentrations in the pulmonary artery, indicating sequestration of fentanyl in the lungs during CPB. The stable fentanyl levels during CPB were thought to imply impaired elimination of fentanyl.	75
Fentanyl	There was a decrease in plasma fentanyl levels far greater than anticipated from the addition of pump prime. Sequestration of fentanyl in the membrane oxygenator was demonstrated.	76

Table continued on following page

TABLE 4–1. STUDIES OF PHARMACOKINETICS AND CARDIOPULMONARY BYPASS *Continued*

Drug	Summary of Authors' Findings	Reference
Fentanyl	Direct in vitro measurements of significant fentanyl absorption by a membrane oxygenator were demonstrated.	77
Gallamine	In the absence of overt signs of renal dysfunction, gallamine disposition in cardiac patients undergoing CPB differed only moderately from that in normal surgical patients.	78
Halothane	The mean temperature-corrected blood/gas partition coefficient for halothane did not change with the inception of hypothermic CPB (because of the offsetting effect of hemodilution), but decreased as the patients were rewarmed (owing to normothermic hemodilution).	79
Isoflurane	Isoflurane was administered through the membrane oxygenator of the bypass pump and resulted in blood levels somewhat lower than expected. The authors felt that their data suggested a possible difference in the uptake of isoflurane into blood from the bypass system compared with the uptake from the lungs.	80
Lidocaine	During CPB the half-life of lidocaine was found to decrease twofold and the volume of distribution to increase twofold. Metabolism of lidocaine was unaltered. These changes in kinetics were attributed to the decrease in concentration of protein-binding sites resulting from dilution of plasma albumin.	81
Lidocaine	Lidocaine kinetics were unchanged 15 minutes and 1 day after CPB, but clearance and volume of distribution were dramatically decreased 3 days after surgery. Lidocaine kinetics returned to base line at 7 days after surgery in most patients, but lidocaine free fraction remained depressed.	6
Midazolam	Used for sedation in the intensive care unit after CPB, midazolam was found to retain "its short duration of action."	82
Nitroglycerin	Nitroglycerin clearance was moderately increased during CPB.	83
Papaverine	The half-life of papaverine during the early hours after CPB was significantly greater than in surgical control patients.	84
Phenoperidine	Phenoperidine was given as a loading dose after induction of anesthesia and was administered by continuous infusion until near the end of surgery. Phenoperidine concentrations transiently decreased with the initiation of CPB. During CPB the phenoperidine levels increased progressively and were greater at the end of bypass than before it. The increase in concentration continued after the termination of CPB. There was no significant absorption of phenoperidine by the CPB pump circuit. Overall, there was no appreciable difference between the measured plasma phenoperidine levels and those predicted using pharmacokinetic data from anesthetized patients undergoing general surgery.	85

TABLE 4–1. STUDIES OF PHARMACOKINETICS AND CARDIOPULMONARY BYPASS *Continued*

Drug	Summary of Authors' Findings	Reference
Piperacillin	Concentrations of piperacillin in plasma during CPB were significantly higher than those in healthy adults given the same intravenous dose. CPB seemed to increase the serum half-life of piperacillin, possibly because of decreased clearance during the operation.	86
Propranolol	Although the last oral dose of propranolol was given approximately 12 hours before CPB, plasma propranolol levels were higher during hypothermia than in the preoperative period, falling to or below control levels after rewarming.	87
Propranolol	Plasma propranolol concentrations fell with the initiation of CPB, but there was no consistent change during CPB. At the end of CPB, plasma propranolol levels began to rise and continued to do so for at least 4 hours, possibly because of equilibration of plasma with lung tissue stores.	88
Sufentanil	After a bolus of sufentanil with the induction of anesthesia, sufentanil plasma levels fell abruptly with the initiation of CPB and seemed to remain unchanged for the remainder of the procedure.	47
Sufentanil	During an exponentially decreasing infusion designed to theoretically maintain a constant plasma sufentanil level, initiation of CPB resulted in an initial decrease in sufentanil concentrations, despite a larger degree of hemodilution as evidenced by the decrease in hematocrit and protein levels. The initial decrease was transient as the plasma levels of sufentanil increased over time as the infusion regimen continued. The inverse relation found between plasma levels and both nasopharyngeal temperature and inflow temperature supported the hypothesis that hypothermia was a major cause of the accumulation of sufentanil during CPB, possibly through inhibition of hepatic drug metabolism and hepatic blood flow.	7
Thiopental	During an exponentially decreasing infusion scheme designed to theoretically maintain a constant plasma thiopental level, total plasma thiopental concentration fell abruptly at the onset of bypass. There was a fall in hematocrit of the same order, suggesting that hemodilution was the cause of the fall in total drug levels. Hemodilution also appeared to cause a decrease in plasma protein binding of thiopental during bypass. At the onset of bypass the unbound plasma thiopental also decreased, but the decrease was smaller than that with total thiopental, probably because of the compensatory effect of the concomitant increase in unbound fraction of drug in plasma. During bypass, the total thiopental level rose gradually but did not reach the prebypass level by the end of surgery. The decrease in unbound thiopental levels was more transient, however, as the prebypass level was reached at the end of bypass.	89

compilation includes several drugs that are not anesthetic drugs, but their perioperative administration is often the responsibility of cardiac anesthetists. Unless indicated otherwise, total (bound + unbound) drug concentrations were measured.

As reflected in Table 4–1, the relation between CPB and pharmacokinetics has attracted a relatively large number of researchers in recent years. Unfortunately many of these investigations have had methodologic shortcomings, and much remains to be learned about the pharmacokinetics of CPB. The abrupt discontinuities that accompany the onset of CPB are difficult to deal with mathematically, and the frequency with which the independent variables (temperature, flow, rate, etc.) change are even more so. When perfusion and ventilation of the lungs are resumed at the end of CPB, washout of drug sequestered in the lungs at the start of bypass can lead to the erroneous conclusion of decreased clearance. Of greatest concern has been the frequent lack of a control group of surgical patients who do not require CPB. In other words, are the drug plasma levels observed during CPB actually different than they would have been without institution of CPB? This is especially important when bolus plus infusion or computerized infusion schemes are utilized; for example, the observation of plasma levels that are higher at the end of bypass than before bypass (Fig. 4–1) does not necessarily imply impaired elimination if the infusion scheme itself is causing the plasma levels to increase.

CPB is conducted in so many variations from surgeon to surgeon, from institution to institution, and even from patient to patient, that attempting to formally describe pharmacokinetics during CPB would probably be a fruitless, if not impossible, task. Moreover, CPB is such a dynamically varying process that to assign a specific value to particular pharmacokinetic parameters "during bypass" is rather misleading, as these parameters are temporally dependent on the phase and duration of CPB. The important pharmacokinetic issue during CPB is whether changes occur that affect the anesthesiologist's ability to maintain appropriate plasma concentrations of drugs administered during the perioperative period. Almost all of the drugs that have been studied demonstrate an abrupt drop in total drug concentrations with the initiation of CPB. Alcuronium, d-tubocurarine, and gallamine are notable exceptions in that the total plasma concentrations of these drugs actually increase with the start of CPB. Interestingly, it may be that the unbound (pharmacologically active) concentrations of drugs that are highly lipid soluble remain relatively unchanged during CPB, as has been shown for alfentanil,[5] lidocaine,[6] and thiopental.[89] It would seem, therefore, that the effects of hemodilution that result from priming the CPB circuit may be partially offset by a redistribution of free drug from the tissues to the bloodstream. After the perturbation in plasma levels that occurs early in CPB, few additional

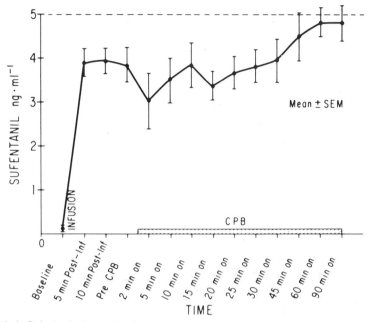

Figure 4–1. Sufentanil plasma levels achieved by a computerized infusion before and during CPB. The set-point sufentanil level was 5 ng • ml^{-+}. *p < .05 versus initial value (5 minutes after start of infusion). (With permission from Flezzani et al: Sufentanil disposition during cardiopulmonary bypass. Can J Anaesth 34:566–569, 1987.)

consistent trends can be identified; plasma levels of most drugs remain relatively constant during CPB, but this depends on the drug, the course of CPB, and the regimen by which the drug is administered.

It has been shown that once CPB exceeds 2 hours, renal tubular membrane dysfunction becomes important,[8] which would presumably impair the postoperative clearance of drugs excreted through renal mechanisms. Thus a second important issue relating to drug disposition and CPB is whether the period of CPB, with its many physiologic implications, results in altered pharmacokinetics during the hours and days after CPB such that modifications in postoperative dosing regimens are required. Digoxin, lidocaine, and midazolam have been investigated in this regard, but, again, modification of "standard" dosing practices was not deemed necessary, which is consistent with the routine clinical experience of most physicians caring for these patients. In the paper by Holley et al.[6] total lidocaine levels were "abnormal" during the first week post CPB, but the free concentrations were within their expected therapeutic range, leading to the conclusion that drug dosing had been appropriate.

CPB is a pragmatic exercise in controlled pathophysiology, which undoubtedly results in a continuous spectrum of changes in drug distribution and elimination, both during and immediately after the bypass period. Such changes have been reported, but evidence to support a priori prophylactic adjustment of drug dosages based on pharmacokinetic grounds has not yet been offered. This later observation is, however, intimately tied to the pharmacodynamic changes that accompany CPB, such as decreased requirement for anesthesia during hypothermia, which render altered drug plasma levels during CPB less significant than they might otherwise be.

ANESTHESIA AND CARDIOPULMONARY BYPASS

The dynamics of drugs used for general anesthesia during CPB have been studied in a limited manner. We have chosen to confine our review to influences on cerebral metabolism, the effect on systemic hemodynamic variables, and the effect of anesthesia on the stress response to CPB.

Influence on Cerebral Metabolism and Flow

Anesthetics affect cerebral metabolism, blood flow, and function during CPB. In addition to anesthetic drugs, there are multiple other factors that affect cerebral blood flow (CBF) during CPB. A study in 67 patients revealed a significant decrease in regional CBF during CPB with nasopharyngeal temperature and $Paco_2$ being the only two significant factors affecting cerebral flow (Table 4–2).[9] CBF and metabolism (expressed as cerebral oxygen consumption [$CMRO_2$]) are temperature dependent and change about 7 per cent per degree Celsius change. Normal $CBF-CMRO_2$ coupling is maintained with decreasing temperature in patients in whom alpha-stat (non–temperature-corrected) blood gas management is conducted. A relatively well matched 30 per cent decrease in CBF and

TABLE 4–2. FACTORS THAT INFLUENCE CBF DURING CPB

Variable	Probability Value
NPT	0.0001
$Paco_2$	0.003
Q	0.06
SVR	0.48
MAP	0.94
Hgb	0.98
Time	0.99

The variables are ranked in order of the greatest influence on cerebral blood flow. The only two variables significant at the $p_2 < .05$ level are NPT and $Paco_2$.

CBF, cerebral blood flow; CPB, cardiopulmonary bypass; NPT, nasopharyngeal temperature; $Paco_3$, partial pressure of arterial carbon dioxide; Q, systemic blood flow; SVR, systemic vascular resistance; MAP, mean arterial pressure; Hgb, hemoglobin; time, aortic cross-clamp time.

$CMRO_2$ occurs at 27° C during nonpulsatile CPB.[10] Hypothermia is thus important in the metabolic control of CBF and the most effective means of depressing cerebral metabolic activity during CPB.

Autoregulation is the ability of the cerebral vasculature to maintain the CBF constant despite wide variations in the mean arterial pressure, thus maintaining a normal oxygen supply-demand ratio. Autoregulation is preserved (i.e., CBF is independent of perfusion pressure changes and dependent on $CMRO_2$) if an alpha-stat management of CO_2 is maintained during hypothermic CPB (Fig. 4–2).[10, 11] CBF is very responsive to changes in $Paco_2$ during CPB in patients anesthetized with high-dose fentanyl (Fig. 4–3)[9, 12]; therefore, it is recommended that $Paco_2$ be maintained at a value of approximately 40 mm Hg (temperature uncorrected). Addition of CO_2 to the pump oxygenator to maintain "normal" Pco_2 when a

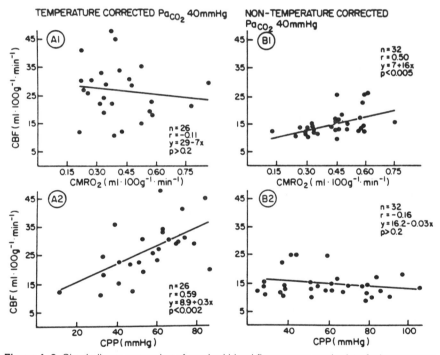

Figure 4–2. Simple linear regression of cerebral blood flow versus cerebral perfusion pressure or cerebral oxygen consumption for temperature-corrected and non–temperature-corrected groups. *Upper panel*: There is no significant correlation between CBF and $CMRO_2$ in the temperature-corrected group (A1), whereas CBF significantly correlates with $CMRO_2$ in the non–temperature-corrected group (B1). *Lower panel*: CBF is significantly correlated with CPP in the temperature-corrected group (A2), whereas CBF is independent of CP in the non–temperature-corrected group (B2). CBF, cerebral blood flow; CPP, cerebral perfusion pressure; $CMRO_2$, cerebral metabolic rate for oxygen. (With permission from Murkin et al: Cerebral autoregulation and flow/metabolism coupling during cardiopulmonary bypass: The influence of $Paco_2$. Anesth Analg 66:825–832, 1987.)

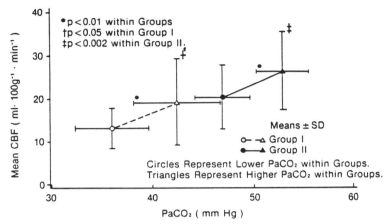

Figure 4–3. CBF response (mean ± SD) to changes in $Paco_2$ in Group I and Group II. CBF increased significantly in both groups in response to changes in $Paco_2$. (With permission from Prough et al: Response of cerebral blood flow to changes in carbon dioxide tension during hypothermic cardiopulmonary bypass. Anesthesiology 64:576–581, 1986.)

temperature correction of blood gases is done results in relative hypercapnia and cerebral vasodilation.[10-12] While not on bypass, a cerebral steal phenomenon has been described in stenosed vessels in which elevated $Paco_2$–induced vasodilation causes shunting of blood from an ischemic area to an area of greater perfusion,[13] and theoretically it is possible that in those patients with stenosed vessels who are temperature corrected for $Paco_2$, cerebral shunting is taking place during CPB. Cerebrovascular responsiveness to Pao_2 is preserved during hypothermic nonpulsatile CPB with alpha-stat management of CO_2.[14] Thus abnormally low Pao_2 will also produce cerebral vasodilation.

The effect of various anesthetic drugs on CBF and $CMRO_2$ is reported in Table 4–3. Although temperature is a more important factor, depth of anesthesia does influence CBF and $CMRO_2$. Anesthesia and hypothermic CPB significantly reduce $CMRO_2$ and CBF from awake values. It is possible to lower CBF and $CMRO_2$ below values seen with high-dose fentanyl anesthesia by giving either thiopental or isoflurane to produce electroencephalographic (EEG) burst suppression.[15] The thiopental group had lower CBF than the isoflurance group, suggesting an uncoupling of CBF to $CMRO_2$ in the isoflurane group. It has been reported that severity of neurologic dysfunction is less in normothermic CPB patients protected with thiopental given in a dose sufficient to produce EEG suppression than in a control "nonprotected" group.[16] Presumably this protective effect is a result of the decrease in metabolic requirements of the jeopardized areas, although this has not been proved. Whether this effect would be seen in hypothermic patients or patients given isoflurane needs to be determined. Also, whether inhalation anesthetics abolish pressure–

flow autoregulation during CPB as they do in normal patients[17] has not been determined. Despite these gaps in our knowledge of CBF and metabolism during CPB, the new information[9-15] enables us to understand and manipulate physiologic and pharmacologic variables during CPB. More neurologic outcome studies are indicated to determine the most appropriate physiologic and anesthetic conditions during CPB.

Influence on Systemic Flow and Temperature

As would be predicted, there are hemodynamic differences between inhalation (halothane) and intravenous (diazepam–fentanyl) anesthesia when administered during CPB. Halothane and isoflurane both tend to reduce the systemic vascular resistance and perfusion pressure[18, 19] compared with intravenous techniques. More vasodilation occurs with isoflurane than with fentanyl.[19] Although these differences in systemic vascular resistance are well documented, they do not seem to influence temperature gradients.[20] Cooling and rewarming were almost identical in patients anesthetized with either fentanyl (100 µg/kg) or halothane (0.5%–1.5%) during bypass. In an early study a tendency toward acidosis was reported in the intravenous anesthesia–treated patients versus those treated with halothane.[18] There have been no systematic studies comparing outcome of inhalation techniques at equal depth to intravenous techniques during CPB as they relate to systemic hemodynamics and patient outcome. Whether acidosis reflects inadequate organ perfusion with ischemic changes in vital tissues needs to be studied. To adequately perform these studies, a definition of equipotent anesthetic depth must be agreed on, or else legitimate dose–response studies must be done.

Stress Response

Characterization of Stress Response

Many investigators have reported a generalized stress response in patients undergoing surgery, and that this response is especially pro-

TABLE 4–3. EFFECT OF ANESTHESIA ON CBF DURING CPB

Drug	Dose	CBF ml/100 g/min	CMRO$_2$ ml/100 gm/min	Temp °C	CO$_2$* mm Hg	Author
Thiopental	17 mg/kg†	8	0.27	26.5	42	Woodcock
Isoflurane	1.1%†	12	0.29	26.6	42	Woodcock
Fentanyl	100 µg/kg	15	0.41	26.8	41	Woodcock
Diazepam/ fentanyl	500/10–20 µg/kg	10	NR	26.3	35	Govier
Awake	—	50	3.0–4.0	37.0	40	Siesjo

NR, not reported.
*Not corrected for temperature
†Given to produce EEG burst suppression.

nounced during CPB. Many organs respond to the stress of CPB by releasing hormones and other vasoactive substances that can be measured in the plasma (Fig. 4–4). For example, the adrenal cortex releases cortisol, the adrenal medulla produces epinephrine, the adrenergic terminals release norepinephrine, and from membrane phospholipids come various prostaglandins. The complement system is also activated through the alternative pathway as well as the classic pathway when blood comes into contact with nonendothelial surfaces. Although there are many other markers of this stress response, we have elected to concentrate on cortisol, catecholamines, and prostaglandins.

The sympathetic nervous system response to CPB has probably best been characterized and has been recently reviewed.[21] The abnormal physiologic state of CPB produces a marked adrenergic response. In the early (1962) experience with CPB, 200 per cent increases in norepinephrine and 1,500 per cent increases in epinephrine were reported.[22] Many subsequent investigators have examined the effect of CPB on the elaboration of endogenous catecholamines.[21, 23–34] The temporal increase in catecholamines in relation to events during CPB in patients undergoing various cardiac operations is shown in Figure 4–5.[33] Epinephrine increased ninefold, peaking while the patients were being rewarmed from induced hypothermia. Peak glucose levels also coincide with rewarming and are probably related to elevated catecholamines (Fig. 4–6).[35] A greater rise generally is reported in epinephrine than in norepinephrine, indicating that the predominant adrenergic response to CPB is a sympathoadrenal (a stress-like) response.[33] This epinephrine response to CPB is also seen in infants and children, demonstrating the similarity of the stress response regardless of age.[36] The greater rise in epinephrine could reflect the greater access of epinephrine to blood, compared with norepinephrine, which tends to stay at its neuronal site of release. To place this

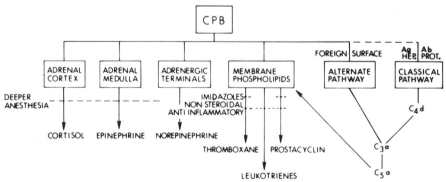

Figure 4–4. Organs and sites of stress-related substances released during cardiopulmonary bypass. Dashed lines indicate methods of reducing the production of stress mediators.

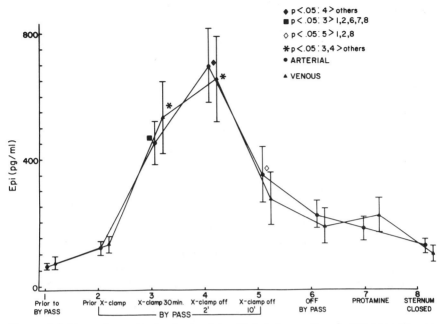

Figure 4–5. Mean plasma levels of epinephrine (Epi) during cardiac anesthesia and surgery. Bars indicate SEM. (With permission from Reves et al: Neuronal and adrenomedullary catecholamine release in response to cardiopulmonary bypass in man. Circulation 66:49–55, 1980.)

catecholamine response in perspective, the epinephrine response to CPB is similar in magnitude to that reported in patients with syncope[37] and in patients with acute myocardial infarction.[38] Values reported for norepinephrine approach the levels seen with strenuous exercise and after caffeine ingestion.[37–39]

The precise causes or mechanisms by which this marked sympathetic response to CPB occurs are not known. The elaboration of endogenous catecholamines probably results from a combination of an increase in the release and a decrease in clearance (metabolism) of catecholamines during CPB. Some factors known to cause a release of catecholamines during CPB include hypothermia, hypotension, hypovolemia, nonpulsatile flow, hemodilution, insulin release, prostaglandin release, myocardial ischemia, hypoperfusion, and renin release. All of these physiologic conditions are associated with a release of endogenous catecholamines in the absence of CPB, and the combination of these stimuli during CPB constitutes a potent stimulus for the release of epinephrine and norepinephrine. Coincident with these causes of an increased production of catecholamines are conditions that contribute to decreased clearance of plasma catecholamines. Clearance of catecholamines occurs primarily in

Blood Glucose

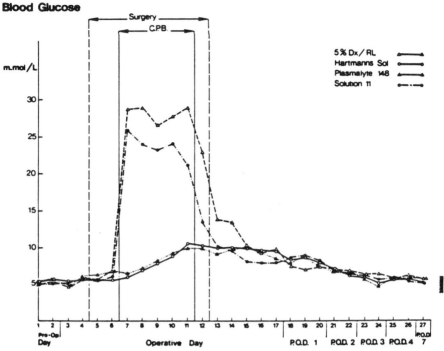

Figure 4–6. Blood glucose concentrations (mmol/L) during and after cardiopulmonary bypass with four pump-priming solutions (mmol/L). CPB, cardiopulmonary bypass; Dx, dextrose; RL, Ringer's lactate; POD, postoperative days. To convert mmol/L to mg/dl multiply by 18. (With permission from McKnight et al: The effects of four different crystalloid bypass pump-priming fluids upon the metabolic response to cardiac operation. J Thorac Cardiovasc Surg 90:97–111, 1985.)

heavily sympathetically innervated organs of the body. Two such organs, lungs and heart, are excluded from the circulation during the time that catecholamines peak during CPB; thus clearance may be reduced. Also, liver perfusion is reduced during CPB, which may account for some reduction in clearance of catecholamines. Particularly important is hypothermia, which slows all enzymatic reactions; therefore, during hypothermic CPB the metabolism of catecholamines, which is enzyme dependent, is reduced in all organs. In addition, metabolic control of the stress response by other hormones is altered by CPB and hypothermia, exacerbating the stress response. For example, hypothermia inhibits release of insulin during CPB, delaying metabolic response to the stress-induced hyperglycemia of CPB. Rewarming during CPB is associated with increased serum insulin concentrations and coincides with a fall in blood glucose levels.[40]

Cortisol rises during CPB and reflects the generalized stress response.

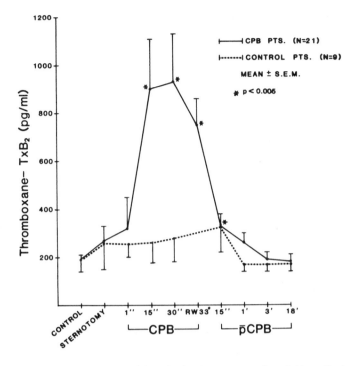

Figure 4-7. Thromboxane concentrations in the two groups of pediatric patients. Note the significantly elevated levels in the CPB group when compared with the control group undergoing palliative surgery without CPB.

It is of interest that although cortisol increases markedly during bypass, the peak cortisol rise in the perioperative period occurs during the first postoperative day.[40] The continuous rise of cortisol and other stress hormones during the first postoperative day indicate that the stress response is not confined solely to the CPB period.

Unlike cortisol, which continues to rise after CPB, but similar to catecholamines and complement, the prostaglandins tend to peak during CPB. There is substantial evidence that prostaglandins are associated with complement activation in the pathophysiologic response to extracorporeal circulation, and represent another marker demonstrating the stress under these conditions. The effects of CPB on prostaglandin metabolism have recently been reviewed.[41] Specifically, thromboxane, the extremely potent bioactive prostaglandin that promotes vasoconstriction and platelet aggregation, has been shown to mediate ischemia and microaggregation during CPB. Prostacyclin is the potent prostaglandin that exerts opposite biologic effects, preserves platelet function and morphology, promotes vasodilation, and may modulate these responses under the same conditions. In adult patients undergoing cardiac surgery, significant increases in thromboxane during CPB have been reported.[42]

The response in prostaglandin production is specifically related to the stresses of CPB. For example, the increase in thromboxane in pediatric patients is much more pronounced in those undergoing CPB than in matched controls having palliative surgical procedures (Fig. 4–7). The evidence suggests that damaged, sequestered platelets synthesize and persistently release physiologically active thromboxane during the period of extracorporeal circulation. Early studies of prostacyclin metabolism and CPB suggested that the increases in prostacyclin synthesis were due to vascular endothelial stimulation by pulsatile and nonpulsatile flow and/or a result of increased thromboxane production.[42] However, in a recent study it was demonstrated that the endogenous release of this prostaglandin may be due to direct mechanical stimulation of vascular endothelial tissue during surgery rather than to the effects of nonpulsatile flow (Fig. 4–8).[43]

The above-mentioned effects of CPB on prostaglandin metabolism appear to be age related. Compared with our adult studies, thromboxane production during CPB is much higher, occurs earlier, and is more

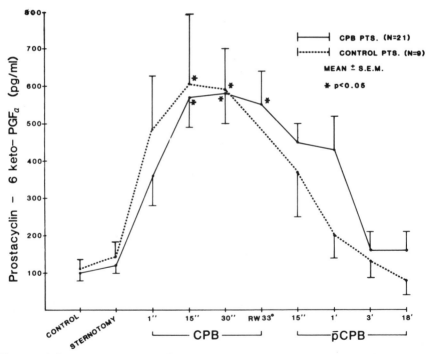

Figure 4–8. Prostacyclin (6-keto-PFG$_1\alpha$) concentrations in two groups of patients (see Fig. 4–7). Note the significant rises in both groups of patients during their operative procedures. There is statistically no difference between groups, except the interval at 1 hour post CPB, where the bypass group was significantly higher compared with the palliative group.

sustained in infants and children (Fig. 4–9).[43] This finding suggests that pediatric patients have greater platelet activation and thromboxane synthesis and release than do adults, or that activation is greater in the young patient because of the greater exposure to non-endothelial artificial surfaces relative to blood volume or size. The highest thromboxane and prostacyclin levels are seen in the youngest patients. This is compatible with the data of Kirklin et al.[44] who reported that the highest levels of complement degradation products occurred in the youngest patients. Both the prostaglandin and complement data support the hypothesis that the damaging effects caused by the stress of CPB may be the greatest in the youngest patients.

The levels of thromboxane and prostacyclin observed during CPB are sufficient to exert pathophysiologic effects on the microcirculation. Because platelet activation and consumption are associated with CPB, and platelet activation is associated with release of thromboxane, there has been substantial investigation into inhibition of this cascade. Specifically, the exogenous administration of prostacyclin and its analogues, all potent inhibitors of platelet aggregation in pharmacologic doses, during CPB has been investigated. Patients given prostacyclin have preserved platelets, decreased activation, and reduced blood loss.[45] This work suggests that the imbalance of the thromboxane-prostacyclin ratio caused by CPB, which may be involved in the tendency toward vasoconstriction and platelet aggregation, can be modified by prostacyclin administration,

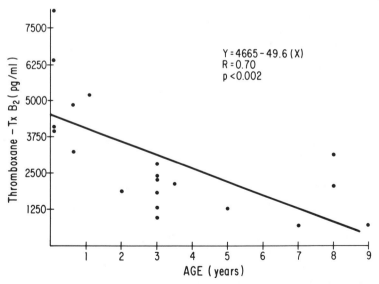

Figure 4–9. Peak thromboxane, corrected for hemodilution, during CPB plotted against patient age. Note that the highest concentrations during CPB occurred in the youngest patients.

resulting in decreased morbidity associated with CPB. Further attempts to link altered prostaglandin metabolism and the pathophysiologic effects of CPB are limited. Although the persistent release of thromboxane is in the range known to exert physiologic responses at the microvascular level, we have demonstrated no correlation between thromboxane production and pulmonary vascular resistance changes in the postoperative period in children.[43] There is a report showing that after reversal of heparin with protamine, a marked pulmonary hypertensive response was associated with increases in thromboxane.[46] However, in general, despite the well-known physiologic effects of prostaglandins and the marked elevations during bypass, no pathologic sequelae have been attributed to them.

Effects of Anesthesia on the Stress Response

A great variety of anesthetic management techniques have been used for patients undergoing cardiac surgery. Several investigations have documented the rise in catecholamines with various anesthetic techniques during CPB in adults[21, 23–33, 36, 47–49] and in children.[36] In general, all anesthetic techniques seem to be accompanied by similar pronounced stress responses during CPB. This reflects the organisms' response to the unusual physiologic conditions that CPB represents and might reflect inadequate depth of anesthesia. Recent studies have, indeed, verified the hypothesis that depth of anesthesia attenuates the stress response to CPB.[19, 47, 49] Two reports in particular support this hypothesis. The first is an investigation comparing enflurane administered during CPB with two different sufentanil administration schemes. Continuous administration of enflurane obtunded the norepinephrine response to CPB (Fig. 4–10)[47] compared with sufentanil (15 μg/kg) given at the beginning of anesthesia. Supplementation of this sufentanil dose with 10 μg/kg at the beginning of CPB also attenuated the initial norepinephrine response to CPB, but as time passed (and presumably as the drug disappeared from the blood) the norepinephrine sparing effect was lost. This supports the hypothesis that adequate blood levels of anesthetic drugs must be present to attenuate the norepinephrine response to CPB. Similarly, in a classic pharmacologic dose–response study,[19] isoflurane diminished the cortisol response to CPB in humans (Fig. 4–11). Isoflurane 2% significantly reduced the cortisol response, compared with patients given only 50 to 58 μg/kg of fentanyl at the beginning of operation. Isoflurane 1% during bypass also attenuated the cortisol response but to a lesser extent than did isoflurane 2%. There appears to be a similar dose effect with opioids as with inhalation anesthesia (Fig. 4–12)[49]; that is, higher plasma levels of sufentanil reduce the norepinephrine response to CPB. These demonstrate that depth of anesthesia does reduce the stress response to CPB.

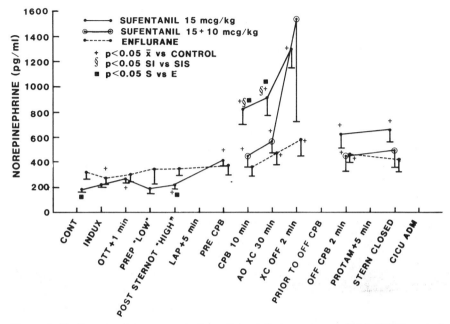

Figure 4–10. Norepinephrine concentrations. Data plotted as mean ± SEM. CONT, control/ base line; INDUX, induction; OTT +1 min, 1 minute after orotracheal intubation; PREP "LOW," lowest systolic pressure during prepping; POST STERNOT "HIGH," highest systolic blood pressure after sternotomy; LAP +5 min, 5 minutes after left atrial line placement; PRE CPB, preceding cardiopulmonary bypass; CPB 10 min, 10 minutes into cardiopulmonary bypass; AO XC 30 min, 30 minutes after the aortic cross-clamp was placed; XC OFF 2 min, 2 minutes after the aortic cross-clamp was removed; PRIOR TO OFF CPB, immediately before coming off cardiopulmonary bypass; OFF CPB 2 min; 2 minutes after coming off cardiopulmonary bypass; PROTAM +5 min, 5 minutes after protamine administration; STERN CLOSED, at sternal closure. (With permission from Samuelson et al: Comparison of sufentanil and enflurane–nitrous oxide anesthesia for myocardial revascularization. Anesth Analg 65:217–226, 1986.)

The mechanisms for this are not clear and have not been investigated, but the concept is logical.

It is not known whether opioids or inhalation agents are more effective in reducing the stress response during CPB. This unanswered question is made difficult by the problem of defining an "equipotent" level of these disparate anesthetic techniques. It is known that the administration of the very high doses of opioids that may be required to block the stress response probably will cause prolonged respiratory depression. Likewise, residual inhalation agents could produce myocardial depression unless they are sufficiently eliminated by means of the pump oxygenator before separation from bypass. It is also known that the anesthetic pharmacokinetic characteristics will influence the duration of stress ablation. For example, the continuous infusion of fentanyl results in higher blood

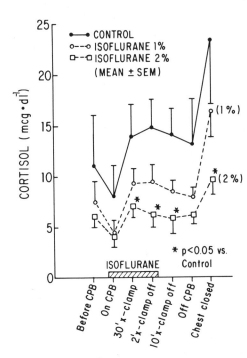

Figure 4–11. Plasma cortisol levels (μg/dl) measured at different times during CABG. CPB, cardiopulmonary bypass; x-clamp, aortic cross-clamp. (With permission from Flezzani et al: Isoflurane decreases the cortisol response to cardiopulmonary bypass. Anesth Analg 65:1117–1122, 1986.)

levels of fentanyl than does the intermittent or "front-end" loading of fentanyl with predictable responses on the stress reaction, that is, continuous infusion is superior to other methods of maintaining a constant, adequate fentanyl level and blocking the release of stress hormones. Also, when alfentanil (short-lasting opioid) is compared with fentanyl (longer-lasting opioid) after cessation of administration of both, the cortisol blocking response is longer lasting with fentanyl than with alfentanil (Fig. 4–13).[50] Interestingly, it has recently been shown that clonidine, an alpha-2 agonist, given to patients before surgery and before CPB, markedly reduced opioid requirements as well as the catecholamine response.[48] Clonidine inhibits adrenergic transmitter release, thus attenuating the adrenergic response to CPB. This nonanesthetic approach to reducing the adrenergic response to CPB merits further study.

Implications of Anesthesia and the Stress Response Period

The implications of increases in plasma catecholamines have been studied more extensively than those of most stress hormones. Epinephrine and norepinephrine both have alpha- and beta-adrenergic agonist properties. Recent studies have shown that during hypothermic CPB, the

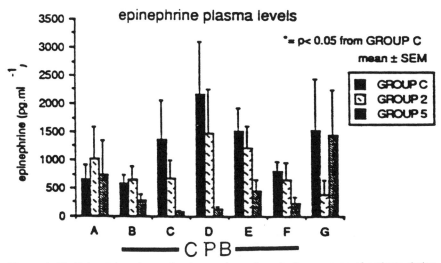

Figure 4–12. Epinephrine plasma levels are shown here in three groups of patients during cardiac anesthesia. Group C received midazolam 0.2 mg/kg and enflurane before cardiopulmonary bypass; Group 2 received the same pre-CPB anesthesia plus continuous infusion of sufentanil (plasma level 2 ng/ml); and Group 5 received sufentanil infusion to a plasma level of 5 ng/ml. Measurement times are A, After sternotomy; B, on CPB; C, 30 min cross-clamped; D, 2 min cross-clamp off; E, 10 min cross-clamp off; F, off CPB; G, chest closed. Note the dose-related effect of sufentanil in diminishing the epinephrine response to CPB. (With permission from Flezzani et al: Effects of a continuous infusion of sufentanil on catecholamine release during cardiopulmonary bypass [abstr]. Society of Cardiovascular Anesthesiologists, 9th Annual Meeting, Palm Desert, Calif, 1987, p. 78.)

alpha-adrenergic response is intact, perhaps even exaggerated.[51, 52] This has been shown using phenylephrine (an alpha-1 agonist) challenge to demonstrate alpha-adrenergic responsiveness, using blood pressure and systemic vascular resistance as the endpoint. Less phenylephrine is required during hypothermic bypass to produce a similar percentage of increase in blood pressure than in the awake patient. This probably represents the additive effect at the alpha-1 receptor of an alpha agonist to the endogenous epinephrine and norepinephrine already present. Other explanations may explain this observation, such as increased numbers of alpha receptors and /or heightened responsiveness of the individual alpha receptor. Whatever the mechanism, it is clear that release of endogenous catecholamines will produce alpha-adrenergic stimulation marked by an increase in systemic vascular resistance and perfusion pressure during bypass. The activity of catecholamines at beta receptors has not been studied during CPB.

In addition to peripheral adrenergic activity, there are myocardial implications for the increased catecholamines during CPB. Table 4–4 lists the most certain physiologic effects. Increases in norepinephrine result in increased mean systemic pressure during aortic cross-clamp-

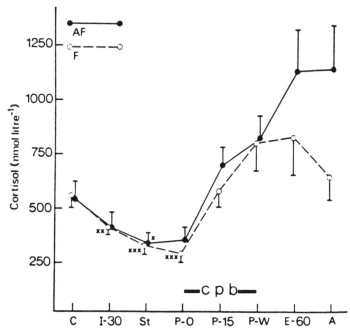

Figure 4–13. Plasma cortisol concentrations in patients anesthetized for coronary artery bypass grafting surgery with continuous infusion of fentanyl or alfentanil (mean + SEM). C, control value after premedication but before induction of anaesthesia; I-30, 30 minutes after initiation of induction of anesthesia; St, maximal sternal spread; P-O, immediately before CPB; P-15, 15 minutes after initiation of CPB; P-W, after rewarming at the end of CPB; E-60, 60 minutes after discontinuation of opiate infusion; A, awakening from anaesthesia. The statistical significance is indicated as follows: O, < .05 between the groups; xx, < .01; xxx, < .001 within the groups. (With permission from Hynynen et al: Continuous infusion of fentanyl or alfentanil for coronary artery surgery. Br J Anaesth 58:1260–1266, 1986.)

ing,[21, 27] which could contribute to cardioplegia washout by way of the noncoronary collateral circulation. The elevated catecholamines could also increase myocardial metabolism and, during reperfusion, cause coronary vasoconstriction and contribute to arrhythmias. The hypothesis that reperfusion of the post-arrested heart with elevated endogenous

TABLE 4–4. IMPLICATIONS FOR MYOCARDIAL PROTECTION OF CATECHOLAMINE RELEASE DURING CARDIOPULMONARY BYPASS

During elective myocardial hypoxia (cross-clamp)
Increased systemic vascular resistance (increased systemic
   pressure = cardioplegia washout)
Increased myocardial metabolism

During myocardial reperfusion
Coronary vasoconstriction
Increased myocardial metabolism
Arrhythmogenesis

catecholamine might contribute to myocardial damage has been examined in 60 patients undergoing coronary artery bypass surgery.[32] Although the heart was exposed to significantly elevated catecholamines (which were taken up by the heart during reperfusion), there was no association of values of epinephrine and norepinephrine uptake with indicators of myocardial damage (CKMB). This lack of deleterious effect may be explained because (a) myocardial protection was sufficient to protect the heart even during reperfusion; (b) norepinephrine and epinephrine were not present in high enough quantities to increase metabolic requirements; or (c) other, much more significant causes of myocardial damage known to be present during cardiac surgery outweigh any lesser effect of the catecholamines. In terms of outcome, it has been shown that postoperative hypertension is mediated by a sympathetic mechanism in many patients. Patients who develop postoperative hypertension are catecholamine responders both during the CPB and during the emergence from anesthesia.[27]

It is thought that cerebral dysfunction after CPB is primarily a result of embolization and ischemia.[53] Either macroembolism[54] or microembolism[55] probably causes much of the neurologic dysfunction seen after CPB. Recent evidence indicates that microembolization does occur in all patients, and the degree of embolism appears to correlate with neurologic dysfunction.[56] The rise in glucose that occurs during CPB is primarily related to whether a glucose prime is used (see Fig. 4–6),[40] but glucose levels certainly are enhanced by the gluconeogenesis produced by elevated catecholamines. There are some indications that elevated glucose can contribute to cerebral ischemia,[57–60] and a recent letter seems to indicate that in children under 1 year of age who undergo circulatory arrest, neurologic outcome is worse in patients with a higher glucose level.[61] These very preliminary data need to be carefully substantiated but tend to support the general idea that high glucose as part of the overall stress response to CPB may have a deleterious impact on neurologic morbidity. It is clear that neurologic dysfunction is related to events during CPB because major vascular patients do not have the same incidence of postoperative neurologic dysfunctions as do cardiac patients.[62]

The release of vasoactive peptides and hormones that constitute the stress response during CPB could contribute to its damaging effects. Figure 4–14 is a schematic illustration of data demonstrating that the duration of CPB relates to morbidity.[44] The longer patients are exposed to CPB, the greater the number of complications. This has been shown particularly for pulmonary and cerebral complications. Certainly the toxicity of CPB is multifaceted, that is, caused by many different factors, and its expression is modulated, at least to some extent, by the patient's susceptibility to the causative factors. It appears that the very young and

CPB TIME-EFFECT

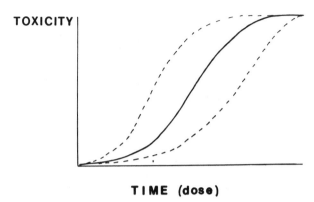

Figure 4–14. There is a relation of TIME (dose) of cardiopulmonary bypass (CPB) to morbidity (TOXICITY) of CPB. We hypothesize that this relation (solid line) may be shifted to the right or left (dashed line). Factors that might shift the curve to the left are extremes of age (elderly or infants) and increased severity of illness. A shift to the left means greater morbidity occurs at less time of exposure. The curve could be shifted to the right by deeper anesthesia, which protects the patient from the damaging effects of CPB.

very old are more susceptible to the damaging effects of CPB. We now advance the hypothesis that anesthesia may *change the susceptibility of a given patient to the deleterious effects of CPB*. This hypothesis is based on the following: (a) it is known that anesthesia can reduce the stress response to CPB in a dose-related manner, and (b) if these vasoactive substances are responsible for the morbidity of CPB, then adequate depth of anesthesia will protect the patient from injury. Organs that might be protected by anesthesia are the heart, brain, kidney, and perhaps other viscera. Of relevance to our hypothesis is a randomized, controlled study in which preterm infants undergoing patent ductus arteriosus ligation were given nitrous oxide and curare with and without fentanyl anesthesia, and hormonal stress responses to surgery and complications were assessed.[63] Major hormonal responses to the stress of this surgery, as indicated by changes in epinephrine, norepinephrine, glucagon, cortisol, glucose, lactate, and pyruvate concentrations, were significantly lower in the groups receiving fentanyl. Further, the fentanyl group had fewer circulatory and metabolic complications postoperatively. This study demonstrates that infants mount a substantial stress response to surgery under anesthesia and that the prevention of this response by fentanyl is associated with improved postoperative outcome. Although the study was done in infants undergoing thoracic surgery without CPB, the attenuation of the stress response by anesthesia is particularly noteworthy. Because CPB is associated with the stress response in children and adults, presumably a similar attenuation of this stress response can be seen with specific anesthetic techniques in which outcome can be improved. Unfortunately no studies have clearly focused on outcome related to depth of anesthesia and mediators of injury during CPB to prove our hypothesis. This is an important area for future investigation.

CONCLUSION

Although all patients requiring CPB are anesthetized, remarkably little information exists to answer the question whether or not specific anesthetics and/or techniques used during CPB are important in determining the patients' postoperative course. Little is known about pharmacokinetics and pharmacodynamics during CPB. Certainly, if high doses of drugs are given during operation, there will be postoperative sequelae such as prolonged ventilation, less hypertension, and perhaps vasoparesis. The question of whether the multitude of vasoactive and perhaps cytotoxic substances released during CPB can be reduced by specific anesthesia, and whether this reduces morbidity, is yet to be answered. We advance the general hypothesis that depth of anesthesia protects against damaging effects of CPB. Related to this are some specific questions: What are the mechanisms by which postoperative morbidity occurs? Is there advantage to blocking or attenuating the stress response? Is one anesthetic or technique superior in accomplishing this? What are the risk and benefits for the use of additional anesthesia during bypass? These and many other questions will be answered as we learn more about appropriate methods of anesthesia during CPB and the pathophysiology of this necessary trespass against normal human biology.

References

1. Holley FO, Ponganis KV, Stanski DR: Effect of cardiopulmonary bypass on the pharmacokinetics of drugs. Clin Pharmacokinet 7:234–251, 1982.
2. Clavey M: Modifications pharmacocinetiques induites par la circulation extacorporelle. Ann Fr Anesth Reanim 5:295–305, 1986.
3. Kamath BSK, Thomson DM: Forum: Administration of drugs during cardiopulmonary bypass. Anaesthesia 35:908–913, 1980.
4. Nussmeier NA, Moskowitz GJ, Weiskopf RB, et al: Anesthetic uptake and elimination via bubble oxygenators: Influence of anesthetic and gas pump flow rates (abstr). Anesthesiology 67:A197, 1987.
5. Hug CC, Burm AGL, de Lange S, et al: Alfentanil pharmacokinetics and protein binding before and after cardiopulmonary bypass (abstr). Proc SCA Fifth Annual Meeting, San Diego, 1983, pp 76–77.
6. Holley FO, Ponganis KV, Stanski DR: Effects of cardiac surgery with cardiopulmonary bypass on lidocaine disposition. Clin Pharmacol Ther 35:617–626, 1984.

7. Flezzani P, Alvis JM, Jacobs JR, et al: Sufentanil disposition during cardiopulmonary bypass. Can J Anaesth 34:566–569, 1987.
8. Suntay GJ, Howie MB, Lingam R, et al: Time related renal consequences of cardiopulmonary bypass (abstr). Anesth Analg 67:S226, 1988.
9. Govier AV, Reves JG, McKay RD, et al: Factors and their influence on regional cerebral blood flow during nonpulsatile cardiopulmonary bypass. Ann Thorac Surg 38:592–600, 1984.
10. Murkin JM, Farrar JK, Tweed A, et al: Cerebral autoregulation and flow/metabolism coupling during cardiopulmonary bypass: The influence of $Paco_2$. Anesth Analg 66:825–832, 1987.
11. Murkin JM: Cerebral hyperperfusion during cardiopulmonary bypass: The influence of $Paco_2$. In Hilberman M (ed): Brain Injury and Protection During Heart Surgery. Boston, Martinus Nijhoff, 1988, pp 47–66.
12. Prough DS, Stump DA, Roy RC, et al: Response of cerebral blood flow to changes in carbon dioxide tension during hypothermic cardiopulmonary bypass. Anesthesiology 64:576–581, 1986.
13. Boysen G, Ladegaard-Pedersen HJ, Henriksen H, et al: The effects of $Paco_2$ on regional cerebral blood flow and internal carotid arterial pressure during carotid clamping. Anesthesiology 35:286–300, 1971.
14. Rogers AT, Stump DA, Prough DS, et al: Cerebrovascular responsiveness to Pao_2 is preserved during hypothermic cardiopulmonary bypass. Anesthesiology 67:A12, 1987.
15. Woodcock TE, Murkin JM, Farrar JK, et al: Pharmacologic EEG suppression during cardiopulmonary bypass: Cerebral hemodynamic and metabolic effects of thiopental or isoflurane during hypothermia and normothermia. Anesthesiology 67:218–224, 1987.
16. Nussmeier NA, Arlund C, Slogoff S: Neuropsychiatric complications after cardiopulmonary bypass: Cerebral protection by a barbiturate. Anesthesiology 64:165–170, 1986.
17. Miletich DJ, Ivankovich AD, Albrecht RF, et al: Absence of autoregulation of cerebral blood flow during halothane and enflurane anesthesia. Anesth Analg 55:100–106, 1976.
18. Norden I: The influence of anaesthetics on systemic vascular resistance during cardiopulmonary bypass. Scand J Thorac Cardiovasc Surg 8:81–87, 1974.
19. Flezzani P, Croughwell N, McIntyre RW, Reves JG: Isoflurane decreases the cortisol response to cardiopulmonary bypass. Anesth Analg 65:1117–1122, 1986.
20. Nieminen MT, Rosow CE, Triantafillou A, et al: Temperature gradients in cardiac surgical patients—a comparison of halothane and fentanyl. Anesth Analg 62:1002–1005, 1983.
21. Reves JG: Adrenergic response to cardiopulmonary bypass. Mt Sinai J Med 52:511–515, 1985.
22. Replogle R, Levy M, DeWall RA, Lillehei RC: Catecholamine and serotonin response to cardiopulmonary bypass. J Thorac Cardiovasc Surg 44:638, 1962.
23. Anton AH, Gravenstein JS, Wheat MW: Extracorporeal circulation and endogenous epinephrine and norepinephrine in plasma, atrium and urine in man. Anesthesiology 25:262, 1964.
24. Tan C, Glisson SN, El-Etr AA, Ramakrishnaiah KB: Levels of circulating norepinephrine and epinephrine before, during and after cardiopulmonary bypass in man. J Thorac Cardiovasc Surg 71:298, 1976.
25. Tan C, Glisson SN, El-Etr AA, Younes SH: Adrenal responses to anesthetics during cardiopulmonary bypass. Cardiovasc Med 3:521, 1978.
26. Hine IP, Wood WG, Mainwaring-Burton RW, et al: The adrenergic response to surgery involving cardiopulmonary bypass, as measured by plasma and urinary catecholamine concentrations. Br J Anaesth 48:355, 1976.
27. Wallach R, Karp RB, Reves JG, et al: Pathogenesis of paroxysmal hypertension developing during and after coronary bypass surgery: A study of hemodynamic and humoral factors. Am J Cardiol 46:559, 1980.
28. Hoar PF, Stone JG, Faltas AN, et al: Hemodynamic and adrenergic responses to

anesthesia and operation for myocardial revascularization. J Thorac Cardiovasc Surg 80:242, 1980.

29. Wood M, Shand DG, Wood AJJ: The sympathetic response to profound hyperthermia and circulatory arrest in infants. Can Anaesth Soc J 27:125, 1980.
30. Balasaraswaaithi K, Glisson SN, El-Etr AA, Azad C: Effect of priming volume on serum catecholamines during cardiopulmonary bypass. Can Anaesth Soc J 27:135, 1980.
31. Stanley TH, Berman L, Green O, Robertson D: Plasma catecholamine and cortisol responses to fentanyl–oxygen anesthesia for coronary-artery operations. Anesthesiology 53:250, 1980.
32. Reves JG, Buttner E, Karp RB, et al: Elevated catecholamines during cardiac surgery: Consequences of reperfusion of the post-arrested heart. Am J Cardiol 53:722–728, 1984.
33. Reves JG, Karp RB, Buttner EE, et al: Neuronal and adrenomedullary catecholamine release in response to cardiopulmonary bypass in man. Circulation 66:49–55, 1980.
34. Feddersen K, Aurell M, Delin K, et al: Effects of cardiopulmonary bypass and prostacyclin on plasma catecholamines, angiotensin II and arginine-vasopressin. Acta Anaesthesiol Scand 29:224–30, 1985.
35. Elliott MJ, Gill GV, Home PD, et al: A comparison of two regimens for the management of diabetes during open-heart surgery. Anesthesiology 60:364–368, 1984.
36. Morgan P, Lynn AM, Parrot C, Morray JP: Hemodynamic and metabolic effects of two anesthetic techniques in children undergoing surgical repair of acyanotic congenital heart disease. Anesth Analg 66:1028–1030, 1987.
37. Robertson D, Johnson GA, Robertson RM, et al: Comparative assessment of stimuli that release neuronal and adrenomedullary catecholamines in man. Circulation 59:637, 1979.
38. Nadeau RA, deChamplain J: Plasma catecholamines in acute myocardial infarction. Am Heart J 98:548, 1979.
39. Cryer PE: Physiology and pathophysiology of the human sympathoadrenal neuroendocrine system. N Engl J Med 303:436, 1980.
40. McKnight CK, Elliott MJ, Pearson DT, et al: The effects of four different crystalloid bypass pump-priming fluids upon the metabolic response to cardiac operation. J Thorac Cardiovasc Surg 90:97–111, 1985.
41. Greeley WJ, Leslie JB, Reves JG: Prostaglandins and the cardiovascular system: A review and update. J Cardiothorac Anesth 4:331–349, 1987.
42. Watkins WD, Peterson MB, Kong DL, et al: Thromboxane and prostacyclin changes during cardiopulmonary bypass with and without pulsatile flow. J Thorac Cardiovasc Surg 84:250, 1982.
43. Greeley WJ, Bushman GA, Kong DL, et al: Effects of cardiopulmonary bypass on eicosanoid metabolism during pediatric cardiovascular surgery. J Thorac Cardiovasc Surg 95:842–889, 1988.
44. Kirklin JK, Westaby S, Blackstone EH, et al: Complement and the damaging effects of cardiopulmonary bypass. J Thorac Cardiovasc Surg 86:845–857, 1983.
45. Fish KJ, Sarnquist FH, Steennis CV, et al: A prospective, randomized study of the effects of prostacyclin on platelets and blood loss during coronary bypass operations. J Thorac Cardiovasc Surg 91:436–442, 1986.
46. McIntyre RW, Flezzani P, Knopes KD, et al: Pulmonary hypertension and prostaglandins after protamine. Am J Cardiol 58:857–858, 1986.
47. Samuelson PN, Reves JG, Kirklin JK, et al: Comparison of sufentanil and enflurane–nitrous oxide anesthesia for myocardial revascularization. Anesth Analg 65:217–226, 1986.
48. Flacke JW, Bloor BC, Flacke WE, et al: Reduced narcotic requirement by clonidine with improved hemodynamic and adrenergic stability in patients undergoing coronary bypass surgery. Anesthesiology 67:11–19, 1987.
49. Flezzani P, Croughwell N, Davis D, et al: Effects of a continuous infusion of sufentanil on catecholamine release during cardiopulmonary bypass (abstr). Society of Cardiovascular Anesthesiologists 9th Annual Meeting, Palm Desert, Calif, 1987, p 78.
50. Hynynen M, Lehtinen AM, Salmenpera M, et al: Continuous infusion of fentanyl or alfentanil for coronary artery surgery. Br J Anaesth 58:1260–1266, 1986.

51. Massagee JT, Kates RA, Reves JG, et al: Effects of preoperative calcium channel blocker therapy on α-adrenergic responsiveness in patients undergoing coronary revascularization. Anesthesiology 67:485–488, 1987.
52. Schwinn DA, McIntyre RW, Hawkins ED, et al: Alpha-1-adrenergic responsiveness during coronary artery bypass surgery: Effect of preoperative ejection fraction. Anesthesiology, in press.
53. Slogoff S, Girgis KZ, Keats AS: Etiologic factors in neuropsychiatric complications associated with cardiopulmonary bypass. Anesth Analg 61:903–911, 1982.
54. Nussmeier NA, McDermott JP: Macroembolization: Prevention and outcome modification. In Hilberman M (ed): Brain Injury and Protection During Heart Surgery. Boston, Martinus Nijhoff, 1988, pp 85–107.
55. Fish KJ: Microembolization: Etiology and prevention. In Hilberman M (ed): Brain Injury and Protection During Heart Surgery. Boston, Martinus Nijhoff, 1988, pp 67–83.
56. Blauth CI, Arnold JV, Schulenberg WE, et al: Cerebral microembolism during cardiopulmonary bypass: Retinal microvascular studies in vivo with fluorescein angiography. J Thorac Cardiovasc Surg 85:668–676, 1988.
57. Lanier WL, Stangland KJ, Schecthauer BW, et al: The effects of dextrose infusion and head position on neurologic outcome after complete cerebral ischemia in primates. Examination of a model. Anesthesiology 66:39–48, 1987.
58. Pulsinelli WA, Brierly JB, Plum F: Temporal profile of neuronal damage in a model of transient forebrain ischemia. Ann Neurol 11:491–498, 1982.
59. Pulsinelli WA, Levy DE, Sigbee B, et al: Increased damage after ischemic stroke in patients with hyperglycemia with or without established diabetes mellitus. Am J Med 74:540–544, 1983.
60. Longstreth WT Jr, Inui TS: High blood glucose level on hospital admission and poor neurologic recovery after cardiac arrest. Ann Neurol 15:59–63, 1984.
61. Steward DJ, DaSilva CA, Flegel T: Elevated blood glucose levels may increase the danger of neurologic deficit following profoundly hypothermic cardiac arrest. Anesthesiology 68:653, 1988.
62. Shaw PJ, Bates D, Cartlidge NEF, et al: Neurologic and neuropsychological morbidity following major surgery: Comparison of coronary artery bypass and peripheral vascular surgery. Stroke 18:700–707, 1987.
63. Anand KJS, Sippell WG, Aynsley-Green A: Randomized trial of fentanyl anaesthesia in preterm babies undergoing surgery: Effects on the stress response. Lancet 1:62–66, 1987.
64. Coniam SW: Alphaxalone infusion during cardiopulmonary bypass. Anaesthesia 35:576–580, 1980.
65. Skacel M, Knott C, Reynolds F, et al: Extracorporeal circuit sequestration of fentanyl and alfentanil. Br J Anaesth 58:947–949, 1986.
66. Polk RE, Archer GL, Lower R: Cefamandole kinetics during cardiopulmonary bypass. Clin Pharmaccol Ther 23:473–480, 1980.
67. Akl BF, Richardson G: Serum cefazolin levels during cardiopulmonary bypass. Ann Thorac Surg 29:109–112, 1980.
68. Miller KW, McCoy HG, Chan KKH, et al: Effect of cardiopulmonary bypass on cefazolin disposition. Clin Pharmacol Ther 27:550–556, 1980.
69. Miller KW, Chan KKH, McCoy HG, et al: Cephalothin kinetics: Before, during, and after cardiopulmonary bypass surgery. Clin Pharmacol Ther 26:54–62, 1979.
70. Storstein L, Nitter-Hauge S, Fjeld N: Effect of cardiopulmonary bypass with heparin administration of digitoxin pharmacokinetics, serum electrolytes, free fatty acids, and renal function. J Cardiovasc Pharmacol 1:191–204, 1979.
71. Walker JS, Shanks CA, Brown KF: Altered d-tubocurarine disposition during cardiopulmonary bypass surgery. Clin Pharmacol Ther 35:686–694, 1984.
72. Lunn JK, Stanley TH, Eisele J, et al: High dose fentanyl anesthesia for coronary surgery: Plasma fentanyl concentrations and influence of nitrous oxide on cardiovascular responses. Anesth Analg 58:390–395, 1979.
73. Bovil JG, Sebel JG: Pharmacokinetics of high-dose fentanyl. Br J Anaesth 52:795–801, 1980.
74. Koska AJ, Romagnoli A, Kramer WG: Effect of cardiopulmonary bypass on fentanyl distribution and elimination. Clin Pharmacol Ther 29:100–105, 1981.

75. Bentley JB, Conahan TJ, Cork RC: Fentanyl sequestration in lungs during cardiopulmonary bypass. Clin Pharmacol Ther 34:703–706, 1983.
76. Koren G, Crean P, Klein J, et al: Sequestration of fentanyl by the cardiopulmonary bypass (CPBP). Eur J Clin Pharmacol 27:51–56, 1984.
77. Rosen DA, Rosen KR, Davidson B, et al: Absorption of fentanyl by the membrane oxygenator (abstr). Anesthesiology 63:A281, 1985.
78. Shanks CA, Ramzan IM, Walker JS, et al: Gallamine disposition in open-heart surgery involving cardiopulmonary bypass. Clin Pharmacol Ther 33:792–799, 1983.
79. Feingold A: Crystalloid hemodilution, hypothermia, and halothane blood solubility during cardiopulmonary bypass. Anesth Analg 56:622–626, 1977.
80. Loomis CW, Brunet D, Milne B, et al: Arterial isoflurane concentration and EEG burst suppression during cardiopulmonary bypass. Clin Pharmacol Ther 40:304–313, 1986.
81. Morrell DF, Harrison GG: Lidocaine kinetics during cardiopulmonary bypass. Br J Anaesth 55:1173–1177, 1983.
82. Lowry KG, Dundee JW, McClean E, et al: Pharmacokinetics of diazepam and midazolam when used for sedation following cardiopulmonary bypass. Br J Anaesth 57:883–885, 1985.
83. Dasta JG, Weber RJ, Wu LS, et al: Influence of cardiopulmonary bypass on nitroglycerin clearance. J Clin Pharmacol 26:165–168, 1986.
84. Kramer WG, Romagnoli A: Papaverine disposition in cardiac surgery patients and the effect of cardiopulmonary bypass. Eur J Clin Pharmacol 27:127–130, 1984.
85. Fischler M, Levron JC, Trang H, et al: Pharmacokinetics of phenoperidine in patients undergoing cardiopulmonary bypass. Br J Anaesth 57:877–882, 1985.
86. Daschner FD, Just M, Spillner G, et al: Penetration of piperacillin into cardiac valves, subcutaneous and muscle tissue of patients undergoing open-heart surgery. J Antimicrob Chemother 9:489–492, 1982.
87. McAllister RG, Bourne DW, Tan TG, et al: Effects of hypothermia on propranolol kinetics. Clin Pharmacol Ther 25:1–7, 1979.
88. Plachetka JR, Salomon NW, Copeland JG: Redistribution of propranolol following cardiopulmonary bypass (abstr). Clin Pharmacol Ther 29:272–273, 1981.
89. Morgan DJ, Crankshaw DP, Prideaux PR, et al: Thiopentone levels during cardiopulmonary bypass. Anaesthesia 41:4–10, 1986.

CHAPTER 5

HEMOSTASIS DURING CARDIOPULMONARY BYPASS

NORIG ELLISON and DAVID R. JOBES

Last year's monograph of the Society of Cardiovascular Anesthesiologists, *Effective Hemostasis in Cardiac Surgery*, was devoted to the subject of this chapter, which reviews that monograph with emphasis on the routine management, the commonly encountered bleeding problems, and the controversial areas.[1]

Many of the problems introduced by applying cardiopulmonary bypass (CPB) to clinical management of heart disease have been successfully addressed. Homologous blood requirements have drastically been reduced, renal dysfunction all but eliminated, and excessive hemolysis is rarely seen. There is general agreement on many practice areas, including (a) preoperative preparation (assessment and treatment) of non-CPB abnormalities of hemostasis and (b) method of inducing, maintaining, and neutralizing heparin anticoagulation. Despite the above, since the beginning of cardiac surgery with CPB in the 1950s, the effects of an artificial circulation on the coagulation system have plagued clinicians and researchers alike. As a result of these effects, many patients do not resume normal hemostasis after neutralization of heparin anticoagulation. This phenomenon is so much a part of cardiac surgery that many have called this abnormal state "normal for these patients," thus focusing on those with sufficient derangements to cause "clinically important" bleeding. This pragmatic categorization may be appealing to clinicians whose primary charge is to care for the patient at hand, but it is somewhat superficial for the intellectual challenge to understanding the basic problem. There have been many attempts to define and solve coagulation problems surrounding CPB. An examination of the body of literature on this subject often results in confusion, especially for the clinician. These frustrations are highlighted by the multiplicity of identifiable contributing patient variables, limitations of investigative tools, and/or conflicting results of investigation and observation. The current reemphasis on transmission of viral illness by way of transfusion suggests that "clinically important bleeding" must now include any need for transfusion and, therefore, be reassessed. A renewed effort is required to improve management of hemostasis.

PREOPERATIVE EVALUATION

The best method for detecting a hemorrhagic diathesis is a properly taken history, and a most important part of that history is the hemostatic response to prior surgical experience or medication. Any bleeding episode should be characterized by severity, site, duration, and presumed cause as well as similar episodes, age at onset of symptoms, and family history. Nearly all significant hereditary disorders of coagulation in an adult patient will be identified at this point. Acquired hemostatic problems may be related to current illness and/or therapy, especially anticoagulants and medication containing aspirin or other platelet-inhibiting drugs. The physical examination may be supportive or add evidence of acquired disorders. Petechiae, ecchymosis, hemarthrosis, or prolonged active bleeding from puncture sites or wounds may be present.

The platelet count, prothrombin time, activated partial thromboplastin time (aPTT), fibrinogen level, and bleeding time have been suggested as a screening hemostatic profile for cardiac surgery. Although no one test or pair of tests is sufficient to make a specific diagnosis or to rule out all potential causes of bleeding, a normal profile and negative history justify the assumption that a hemorrhagic diathesis is not present. The work of Salzman et al.[2] suggests that incorporation of a factor VIII:vWF assay into the profile is highly desirable. In their study, the preoperative level of Factor VIII:vWF correlated highly with postoperative blood loss.

The practice of ordering any routine battery of tests is certain to be questioned in this era of cost containment. At the University of Pennsylvania, in the last 6,000 open heart operations, one previously undiagnosed very mild Factor IX deficiency was first detected by a prolonged aPTT on a screening profile. Does this justify such a routine practice? Alone, it probably does not. However, the ability to discount a preexisting hemorrhagic diathesis as a cause of excessive bleeding post bypass is most reassuring in managing those patients who are bleeding excessively. With a negative history and a normal screening profile that assumption is, indeed, valid. Further, the values obtained with this profile will serve as base line figures to which values obtained intraoperatively can be compared (e.g., a decrease in platelet count of 200,000 to 50,000 indicates a change in the wrong direction). Obviously any abnormality discovered in the preparatory phase should result in definitive evaluation and correction. The vast majority of such problems are successfully handled in the elective patient population.

Unfortunately the percentage of nonelective cardiac surgical patients for whom delays are impossible and who at the same time are at increased risk of hemostatic derangement is *increasing!* Antiplatelet therapy is often used in patients with angina who may require urgent surgery if they become unstable. Patients who have unsuccessful percutaneous transluminal coronary artery angioplasty or experience complications of that procedure may require immediate surgery and may have previous or ongoing heparin administration. Fibrinolytic therapy of acute coronary thrombosis is becoming more commonplace, and surgery may be required if it fails. Operations performed less than 12 hours after streptokinase have resulted in three times the blood loss with the additional requirements for epsilon-aminocaproic acid (EACA), cryoprecipitate, fresh frozen plasma, and fibrinogen.[3] These situations dictate that we can only prepare and apply therapeutic intervention later in the course of surgery, usually after the adverse effects of CPB have been added. A high index of suspicion, a thorough understanding of new techniques, immediate meaningful laboratory assessment, and promptly available specific treatment must be applied for successful management.

HEPARIN ANTICOAGULATION AND ITS NEUTRALIZATION

Extracorporeal circulation systems are made of materials that stimulate the coagulation process to such an extent that inhibition is necessary to prevent pathologic thrombus formation. Heparin has been used for this purpose since the introduction of CPB. Heparin appears to be highly satisfactory because it is specific, has few side effects, has virtually no time limit, and an antidote is available. The only previous contraindication for heparin use in CPB, heparin-induced thrombocytopenia, is now successfully managed with platelet-inhibiting drugs.[4] The most significant achievements in heparin use since the advent of CPB have been identification of variable patient response to dose, the effect of hypothermia in slowing heparin elimination, and the ability to monitor and maintain satisfactory anticoagulation with more precision.

The ability to individualize heparin therapy during cardiac surgery required a test that provided accuracy and rapidly available results. Two "bedside" methods, protamine titration and activated coagulation time (ACT), evolved. Manual and automated versions for both methods are currently used.[5]

Sufficient heparin is necessary to prevent invisible low-grade coagulation as well as gross thrombosis. Identification of a minimum safe level of anticoagulation would be ideal. The systematic identification of thrombus formation and depletion of coagulation factors in humans as a result of artificial circulation when using heparin can be found in the reports of long-term extracorporeal membrane oxygenation (ECMO).[6] The ACT was maintained between 170 and 240 seconds by protocol in an attempt to balance risks of excessive versus inadequate anticoagulation. At least 9 of 22 patients had evidence of thrombosis. Although short-term use of CPB for surgery may not be exactly the same as the ECMO perfusions, it is similar and strongly suggests that 170 to 240 seconds will be inadequate to prevent thrombus formation at some point in CPB.

Our observations using a manual protamine titration suggested that no visible evidence of coagulation occurred when the test showed ≥30 µg/ml (simultaneous Hemochron ACT was always ≥300 seconds).[7] Bull et al.[8] made the same observation (i.e., no visible clot if manual ACT was ≥300 seconds but recommended a minimum value of 480 seconds.[9] Young et al.[10] observed fibrin monomer formation in primates when the ACT ≥326 seconds. The appearance of accumulated debris on oxygenator filters by electron micrographs correlated with ACT levels at which monomer was detected. Fibrin monomer could not be demonstrated in five pediatric patients whose ACT was 450 seconds or greater. Young et al.[10] therefore recommended a 400-second minimum ACT in humans. Two groups have utilized a fixed heparin protocol and followed the ACT. Culliford et al.[11] found no evidence of fibrin deposition on arterial filters by scanning electron microscopy in six patients whose ACT ranged as low as 249 seconds. Metz and Keats,[12] using a similar protocol, were unable to detect visible thrombus in the pump system after CPB in 42 patients where the lowest ACT ranged from 234 to 400 seconds. They compared chest tube drainage with ACT in these as well as in more than 100 other patients and found no correlation. They concluded that significant coagulopathy did not occur within that range of ACT. The minimum values most often used for maintenance of anticoagulation, 480 seconds (Bull et al.[8]) and 400 seconds (Young et al.[10]), have been considered safe margins for error between absolute minimum and unwarranted excess. As such, they must be viewed as guides for prudent excess until more accurate data are obtained.

What has been the impact of more precise control of anticoagulation for CPB? Mammen et al.[13] pointed out that there is a clear difference in reports of extensive fibrinolysis after CPB published before 1970 compared with more recent papers, in which only slightly elevated fibrin split products were observed. Borderline or inadequate anticoagulation may result in low-grade activation of coagulation and produce secondary fibrinolysis. Therefore, the observations of Mammen et al.[13] may be explained by the introduction and widespread acceptance by the mid-1970's of the concept of individualized heparin titration to a defined endpoint, resulting in more uniform anticoagulation. This point has been made by Bull,[14] who stated, "The major risk is not too much heparin but too little, with the precipitation of disseminated intravascular coagulation (DIC)." The major emphasis on risk of insufficient heparin must be tempered, however, to also avoid unwarranted excess. It must also be remembered that the dose of heparin dictates the dose of protamime. Monitoring and titration have usually caused a reduction in total heparin dose and, therefore, protamine. Decreased doses of protamine have been associated with reduced postoperative bleeding.[15]

Prompt heparin neutralization after CPB is required for effective hemostasis. Protamine is almost exclusively utilized. Protamine is highly efficient in this regard but, unlike heparin, produces significant undesirable effects. Though complement activation is substantial during CPB, a marked increase occurs immediately after protamine administration. Systemic arterial hypotension during protamine administration is common and can be profound. Morbidity and mortality have resulted from ill-defined (allergic?) protamine reactions.[16] Fortunately they are uncommon in adults and have not been observed in infants. Because neutralization of heparin by protamine depends on the amount of circulating drug (as opposed to heparin effect), an assessment of circulating heparin level is a more precise guide to protamine dose. Also, precise measurement of plasma volume is necessary to match heparin to protamine exactly. Neither assessment is easily performed and approximations for both are used. Virtually all recommendations for arriving at a neutralizing dose result in an excess of protamine. The clinical risk of inadequate coagulability is currently thought to exceed any ill-defined negative influence of a modest surplus of protamine. An additional rationale for an overabundance of circulating protamine is "heparin rebound." Such later reappearance of circulating heparin has been documented but is extremely variable in reported incidence and is seldom identified as a reason for excessive bleeding postoperatively.[17] If suspected, a one-step protamine titration may detect it. More commonly, a small dose of additional protamine is simply administered empirically. Further research in this area should lead to a more uniformly applied protamine dosage schedule than currently exists and/or the development of a better antidote.

Alternatives to heparin and protamine are few and of limited clinical value and experience. Absolute removal of a major element in the coagulation mechanism has been reported (defibrinogenation with ancrod).[18] This technique has significant restrictions at this time and is limited in its application. The lack of development of suitable alternatives to heparin and protamine may reflect general acceptance and satisfaction with these drugs, but the more widely recognized serious side effects of protamine and the knowledge that heparin is not always effective may stimulate discovery of new and better techniques.

ACHIEVING HEMOSTASIS AFTER CPB

Approximately 10 per cent to 20 per cent of patients exhibit inadequate hemostasis of varing duration and severity requiring treatment that includes multiple transfusions of blood products.

Table 5–1 lists the most frequently used successful therapeutic modalities to achieve hemostasis after CPB, and from them can be inferred the common identifiable causes of bleeding. However, much confusion and controversy exist at this point. A clear uniform clinical definition of "excessive" or "abnormal" bleeding to guide observations, decision making, and experimentation is lacking. Although defining "excessive" is arbitrary, we recommend one approach. Table 5–2 is a well-tested protocol that defines excessive as the need for reoperation. Patients who meet the levels indicated will also have been in need of blood products for treatment. The effects of testing and type of treatment could be assessed against such a table as well and be a more reliable estimate of the incidence of problematic bleeding after CPB.

The following potential causes of excessive bleeding are found to varying degrees in virtually all patients after CPB: fibrinolysis, decreased Factors V and VIII, decreased fibrinogen, decreased plasminogen, decreased number of platelets (thrombocytopenia), decreased function of platelets, and complement activation. Standard clinical laboratory assessments of the coagulation mechanism are virtually all abnormal compared with the range of values obtained from healthy people. Highly refined laboratory research techniques have uncovered more abnormalities. The emphasis of much recent research has focused on the platelet. This complex vital hemostatic component has been carefully and exhaustively examined. In vitro analysis of platelet function under many conditions has been performed. There is general agreement that platelets become structurally, functionally, and quantitatively abnormal as a result of CPB. Many drugs and conditions are now known to alter platelet function, and because more than one of these exist simultaneously in most CPB patients, it is almost surprising that effective hemostasis is

TABLE 5–1. HEMOSTATIC TREATMENT MODALITIES AFTER CPB

Sutures
Protamine
Fresh whole blood*
Platelets
Plasma†
Avoidance of hypertension
Patience, persistence, and/or prayer

*Recommended by some, especially in infants. Logistical considerations dictate that fresh whole blood is unlikely ever to be widely used.
†Plasma is listed because of its prevalent use, although the justification for this widespread use is surely lacking.

TABLE 5-2. CHEST DRAINAGE CRITERIA FOR REENTRY

Preoperative Weight (kg)	Chest Drainage Indicating Reoperation				
	Hourly Amount (ml h⁻¹) No. of Successive Hrs.			Total Amount (ml) Hour No.	
	1	2	3	4	5
5.0	70	60	50	120	130
6.0	70	60	50	130	155
7.0	70	60	50	150	180
8.0	90	70	50	175	200
9.0	90	80	60	195	230
10.0	100	90	65	220	260
12.0	130	100	80	260	300
14.0	150	120	90	300	360
16.0	170	140	100	350	400
18.0	195	150	120	390	460
20.0	200	175	130	450	520
25.0	270	220	160	540	650
30.0	325	260	195	650	770
35.0	380	300	230	760	990
40.0	430	350	260	800	1,035
45.0	500	400	300	975	1,150
50.0	500	400	300	1,000	1,200

(From Kirklin JW, Barratt-Boyes BG: *Cardiac Surgery*. New York, Churchill Livingstone, 1986, p. 159. Reproduced with permission of the authors and publisher.)

ever achieved. There is no clinically useful assessment of platelet function that is agreed to accurately predict which patient will undergo excessive bleeding. Prophylactic platelet transfusion is therefore not warranted. Clinicians are likely to use empiric platelet transfusion in post-CPB bleeding because of today's increased focus on platelet abnormalities. We lack the ability to be certain that the observed bleeding is, in fact, due to problems with platelets. Platelet transfusion, for reasons of suspected or even measured "platelet dysfunction," must be viewed with some skepticism. Lambert et al.[19] restored hemostasis in bleeding patients after CPB without platelet administration by using EACA and cryoprecipitate. This management succeeded despite documented platelet dysfunction in all patients in this large series. There is in vitro evidence that cryoprecipitate helps to restore platelet function, which may explain these results. Nonetheless, the administration of cryoprecipitate guarantees multiple donor exposure.

Preserving endogenous platelets would seem to be better than current modes of therapy. Membrane oxygenators are less damaging to platelets than bubble oxygenators.[20] Inhibition or restoration of platelet function with drugs has shown promise, and we may soon see positive results of widespread clinical trials with iloprost, desmopressin acetate, or dipyridamole.[3, 5, 20]

Lack of benefit and increased risks associated with prophylactic administration of platelets and fresh frozen plasma have led most, if not all, experts to caution against these and other forms of empiric or "shotgun" therapy. The alternative is to use a battery of specific tests with immediate results that can be serially repeated. This ideal is almost impossible to achieve in the circumstances surrounding an acutely bleeding patient. This represents exactly the dilemma that confronts clinicians today and results in the prevalent empiric management. A major challenge that remains is to bring the laboratory closer to the clinical setting with respect to both test specificity and rapidity of results.

An alternative to blood component therapy for bleeding after CPB is to administer freshly drawn whole blood. This practice is largely limited to infants, in whom extreme dilution or destruction of most clotting factors is predictable. The use of fresh whole blood will rapidly restore the hemostatic system and minimize multiple-donor exposure. The availability of sufficient donors is possible and practical in infants.

The future will probably produce at least partial solutions to the problem of altered hemostasis. Less reactive artificial surfaces bonded with heparin and readily titratable platelet inhibitors will be the earliest modalities likely to reach the clinician. Desmopressin has a beneficial effect, but its precise role awaits definition. Currently, meticulous attention to preoperative hemostatic evaluation, ensuring an adequate response to pre-CPB heparin administration, intra-CPB maintenance of adequate heparin effect, and post-CPB protamine neutralization of heparin are the essential first steps in securing effective hemostasis. Legitimate indications for platelets, fresh frozen plasma, or other specific therapeutic modalities require more precise and timely evaluations of hemostasis.

References

1. Ellison N, Jobes D (eds): Effective Hemostasis in Cardiac Surgery. Philadelphia, WB Saunders, 1988.
2. Salzman EQ, Weinstein MJ, Weintraub RM, et al: Treatment with desmopressin acetate to reduce blood loss after cardiac surgery. N Engl J Med 314:1402–1406, 1986.
3. Lee KF, Mandell J, Rankin JS, et al: Immediate versus delayed coronary grafting after streptokinase treatment. J Thorac Cardiovasc Surg 95:216–222, 1988.
4. Addonizio VP Jr, Fisher CA, Jenkin BA, et al: Iloprost (ZK36374), a stable analogue of prostacyclin preserved platelets during simulated extracorporeal circulation. J Thorac Cardiovasc Surg 899:926–933, 1985.
5. Jobes DR, Schwartz AJ, Ellison N, et al: Monitoring heparin anticoagulation and its neutralization. Ann Thorac Surg 31:161–166, 1981.
6. Heiden D, Mielke CH, Rodvein R, et al: Platelets, hemostasis, and thromboembolism during treatment of acute respiratory insufficiency with extracorporeal membrane oxygenation. J Thorac Cardiovasc Surg 70:644–655, 1975.
7. Jobes DR, Bikhazi G, Ellison N: Rapid assessment of heparin anticoagulation and

reversal. Abstracts of Scientific Papers, American Society of Anesthesiologists Annual Meeting, 1976, p 437.

8. Bull BS, Korpman RA, Huse WM, et al: Heparin therapy during extracorporeal circulation, I. J Thorac Cardiovasc Surg 69:674–684, 1975.

9. Bull BS, Huse WM, Brauer FS, et al: Heparin therapy during extracorporeal circulation, II. J Thorac Cardiovasc Surg 69:685–689, 1975.

10. Young JA, Kisker CT, Doty DB: Adequate anticoagulation during cardiopulmonary bypass determined by activated clotting time and the appearance of fibrin monomer. Ann Thorac Surg 26:231–240, 1978.

11. Culliford AT, Gitel SN, Starr N, et al: Lack of correlation between activated clotting time and plasma heparin during cardiopulmonary bypass. Ann Surg 193:105–111, 1981.

12. Metz S, Keats A: ACT values during cardiopulmonary bypass and patient outcome. Society of Cardiovascular Anesthesiologists, 10th Annual Meeting, 1988, p 146.

13. Mammen EF, Koets AS, Washington BC, et al: Hemostasis changes during cardiopulmonary bypass. Semin Thromb Hemost 11:281–292, 1985.

14. Bull BS: Heparin anticoagulation (letter). Ann Thorac Surg 29:204, 1980.

15. Guffin AV, Dunbar RW, Kaplan JA, et al: Successful use of a reduced dose of protamine after cardiopulmonary bypass. Anesth Analg 55:110–113, 1976.

16. Morel DR, Zapol WM, Thomas SJ, et al: $C5_a$ and thromboxane generation associated with pulmonary vaso- and bronchoconstriction during protamine reversal of heparin. Anesthesiology 66:597–604, 1987.

17. Jobes DR, Schwartz AJ, Ellison N: Heparin rebound (letter). J Thorac Cardiovasc Surg 82:940–941, 1981.

18. Zulys VJ, Glynn MFX, Teasdale S, et al: Ancrod as an alternative to heparinization during cardiopulmonary bypass. Society of Cardiovascular Anesthesiologists, 9th Annual Meeting, 1987, p 81.

19. Lambert CJ, Marengo-Rowe AJ, Leveson JE, et al: The treatment of postperfusion bleeding using epsilon-aminocaproic acid, cryoprecipitate, fresh frozen plasma, and protamine sulfate. Ann Thorac Surg 28:440–444, 1979.

20. Teoh KH, Christakis GT, Weisel RD, et al.: Blood conservation with membrane oxygenators and dipyridamole. Ann Thorac Surg 44:40–47, 1987.

CHAPTER 6

EMERGENCE FROM CARDIOPULMONARY BYPASS: Controversies about Physiology and Pharmacology

JOHN R. MOYERS and JOHN H. TINKER

Emergence from cardiopulmonary bypass (CPB) involves management of a patient who has, in essence, sustained a cardiac arrest. The anesthesiologist should understand this and be prepared to resuscitate the patient during this crucial change in cardiopulmonary physiology. Some aspects are different in this situation from other cardiac arrests. The patient has been provided with CPB with its accompanying organ perfusion plus some control of physiology and metabolism. Efforts have been made toward myocardial preservation. The cardiac operating room team has had time to plan and prepare for separation from bypass. The airway has been secured and the anesthesiologist is prepared to ventilate the patient with oxygen. The primary focus can therefore be on cardiac function, with emergence from bypass occurring only when the entire team is ready. These aspects (Table 6–1) can be used to advantage to create as

TABLE 6–1. FACTORS TO CONSIDER IN PREPARATION FOR EMERGENCE FROM CARDIOPULMONARY BYPASS

1. Body temperature
2. Laboratory data
3. Depth of anesthesia
4. Ventilation
5. Cardiac rhythm
6. Function of monitors
7. Preparedness of the surgical field
8. Circulatory support drugs and mechanical devices
   a. Inotropes
   b. Vasodilators
   c. Mechanical assist devices

safe and controlled an atmosphere as possible to achieve satisfactory emergence from bypass (i.e., a return to reliance on the patient's own heart and lungs). This chapter discusses those features important in satisfactory emergence from CPB, especially areas in which controversy exists.

TEMPERATURE

Patients are usually cooled during CPB to levels of moderate hypothermia (25°–30° C). Before separation from bypass, the patient must be rewarmed. The temperature of highly perfused, accessible tissues such as the nasopharynx and the esophagus should reach 37° C. Rectal temperature, as a measure of more peripheral temperature, should be near or above 35° C. Palpation of the patient's head, shoulders, and hands at this time may also be helpful in assessing the extent of rewarming. Some anesthesiologists will want to see the temperature of the great toe at 30° C or above; others will monitor urine temperature. Some investigators have found urine temperature to coincide with blood temperature,[1] whereas others have found it to represent temperature areas of intermediate blood flow.[2] Although bladder temperature is considered reliable by some as an indication of temperature,[3] urine flow may affect its temperature in the bladder. High urine flow, from a warm kidney, may prematurely convince the anesthesiologist that the periphery is adequately rewarmed. During sternal closure, temperature may decrease such that a 2° to 3° C "afterdrop" has occurred by the time the patient has been transferred to the intensive care unit.[4–7] Instability in cardiac rhythm and shivering with markedly increased $\dot{v}o_2$ are among unwanted effects of this "afterdrop" type of hypothermia.

Nitroprusside-induced vasodilation combined with increased pump flows during rewarming on bypass may lessen postbypass temperature drop.[5, 8] Vasodilation caused by nitroprusside must be balanced against necessary coronary perfusion pressure by increasing pump flows if this method of amelioration of postbypass temperature drop is to be helpful. Noback and Tinker[5] postulated that during rewarming, constricted vascular beds may not dilate, and therefore warming is incomplete. The temperature drop later is thought to be caused by later redistribution of heat within the body, presumably as resumption of pulsatile flow now opens up relatively colder vascular beds. Some investigators have advocated use of pulsatile flow on bypass during rewarming to increase capillary flow within cold tissue beds,[9, 10] particularly muscle.[8, 11] Pulsatile flow may be accomplished either by a pulsatile flow–generating device incorporated into the pump oxygenator[9] or by partially occluding venous return to the pump and allowing left ventricular ejection of blood during partial bypass.[10] Although controversial, better peripheral flow conditions during pulsatile bypass may be due to greater mechanical energy input. In contrast, a study by Singh et al.[12] found neither more complete nor faster rewarming with a pulsatile flow pattern. Heating blankets may be ineffective in this situation. Burns are always a possibility with such devices, especially because if the blanket does not seem effective, the tendency is to turn up its temperature. In adults increases in room temperature probably have little effect once afterdrop has occurred, but may be helpful in prevention. Use of heated, humidified gases after bypass to prevent hypothermia is controversial. Caldwell et al.[13] prevented a drop in temperature after bypass in a study of five patients with heating (46°–7° C) and humidifying inspired gases.[13] Conversely, Ralley et al.[14] found no advantage with use of heated humidifiers. The latter study concluded that it was preferable to warm fully at conclusion of bypass rather than rely on any ability to add heat to the patient later. Finally, it is important that communication among the team occur so that the end of surgical repair coincides with a thoroughly warmed patient.

LABORATORY DATA BEFORE EMERGENCE FROM BYPASS

The patient's metabolic status should be assessed and abnormalities corrected before conclusion of bypass. Arterial and mixed venous blood gas measurements should be obtained, with special attention paid to pH. Most cardiac teams would like to see the hematocrit between 20 and 25 per cent. Serum potassium, sodium, and ionized calcium should be checked. Serum glucose is often elevated at the end of bypass, presumably because elevated catecholamines stimulate hepatic glycogenolysis. The serum glucose level usually returns toward normal in the first few hours in the intensive care unit. This fact must be weighed against the potential detrimental effects of hyperglycemia on cerebral ischemia, but administration of insulin is seldom warranted just for the purpose of lowering blood glucose.

ANESTHETIC REQUIREMENT

During rewarming the patient rapidly loses the anesthetic effect of hypothermia because of the large cerebral flow of warmed blood. At this point, preventing and/or treating awareness must be weighed against the possibility of circulatory depressant effects of anesthetic drugs. Additional drugs for amnesia, such as scopolamine, benzodiazepines (especially lorazepam), or ketamine, may be used. Unless a narcotic infusion technique has been in use throughout bypass, additional narcotics will probably be needed for analgesia. The circulatory depressant effects of various intravenous drugs must be taken into account, and volatile anesthetic agents either discontinued or inspired concentrations greatly decreased. If isoflurane has been in use during bypass, administered by way of the oxygenator, most will be eliminated if discontinued ten minutes before termination at usual oxygenation gas flows (Fig. 6–1).[15] This is a time to check that the vaporizer on the CPB machine has been turned off, as well as the vaporizers on the anesthesia machine. In addition, any vasodilators (or vasopressors) administered during bypass and still in use should be reassessed. The anesthesiologist should anticipate which anesthetic will be used when needed after discontinuation of bypass.

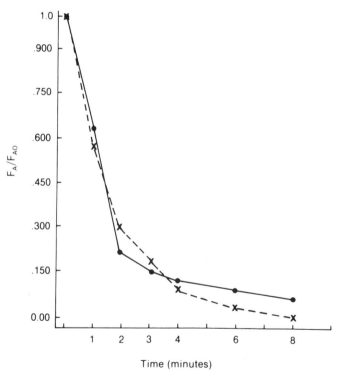

Time (minutes)

Figure 6–1. Actual and predicted one-compartment model of isoflurane washout curves. Key: F_A = measured isoflurane concentration; F_{AO} = baseline measured isoflurane concentration; X (dashed line) = predicted isoflurane F_A/F_{AO} ratios for patient; ● (solid line) = actual isoflurane F_A/F_{AO} ratios for patient. (From Price SL, et al.: Isoflurane elimination via a bubble oxygenator during extracorporeal circulation. J Cardiothoracic Anes 2:41, 1988, with permission.)

VENTILATION

As with any cardiopulmonary resuscitation, one cannot proceed until the airway and ventilation are established. The anesthesiologist must achieve bilateral lung inflation with oxygen through a patent endotracheal tube. Pulmonary compliance should be checked and adequate tidal volume ensured. Lung deflation should be assessed with a high index of suspicion for bronchospasm or prolonged deflation. The left lung, especially the lower lobe, should be checked for atelectasis. If the internal mammary artery has been used, the adequacy of its length should be again checked. Does the patient have a pneumothorax? Is blood or fluid trapped in either hemithorax? Vigorous ventilation and Valsalva maneuver may be helpful to remove trapped air in the left side of the heart. Adequacy of oxygenation and carbon dioxide removal should be assessed later in a more quantitative manner after separation from bypass and pulmonary blood flow has been restored.

CARDIAC RHYTHM

A cardiac rhythm that can be expected to produce a reasonable output must be obtained. In preparation, a properly functioning defibrillator and a pacemaker must be available, the latter preferably of the atrioventricular (AV) sequential type. Is the patient likely to need atrial, ventricular, or AV pacing? Are any antiarrhythmic drugs anticipated? Because rhythm changes occur so frequently at the end of bypass, for many reasons, it is often unwise to rush in early with large doses of antiarrhythmic drugs, especially immediately before termination of bypass. In contrast, use of a pacemaker-driven rhythm or higher rate is common before attempting separation.

Rate, rhythm, and conduction should be assessed and abnormalities corrected, if possible, while the patient is still on bypass. Normal sinus rhythm may return spontaneously after cross-clamp removal. Often normal conduction evolves after varying degrees of AV dissociation. The most common sequence of events is development of ventricular fibrillation after cross-clamp removal, requiring direct current defibrillation. Sustained ventricular fibrillation in this period will increase myocardial oxygen consumption and introduce the possibility of left ventricular distention, if a functioning left ventricular vent is not in place. For adults in ventricular fibrillation, 2.5 to 40.0 J is usually sufficient. One should begin with the lowest power setting expected to work because myocardial damage can occur. If defibrillation is unsuccessful, one should address the following issues[16, 17]: Is the patient's temperature too low? Are hypoxia and/or acidosis involved? Is there coronary obstruction with air or by some other mechanism? Is the defibrillator faulty? Is the patient hypotensive (mean systemic blood pressure less than 50 mm Hg)? Lake et al.[17] reported that patients with valvular disease were more difficult to defibrillate than those with coronary disease, but that this was not related to estimated ventricular weight or wall thickness as postulated by others. This study[17] is the most extensive modern human study to date of this important subject, and it emphasizes the use of lower power settings than are commonly employed.

Bradycardia during emergence from bypass is usually best treated with electrical pacing; it is difficult to titrate to a desired heart rate with atropine or isoproterenol. Sinus tachycardia at the end of bypass may slow as the patient is taken off bypass and the heart filled during venous outflow line occlusion. Tachycardia might also be a sign of "light" anesthesia, but this may not be the best moment to drastically deepen it. In the case of a patient undergoing coronary bypass grafting, tachycardia may not be ominous and probably does not need immediate treatment because major coronary obstructions have been bypassed. Also, this previously globally ischemic heart will now often have very *rate-dependent output*. If sinus tachycardia is persistent and requires treatment after separation is successful and output known, small doses of esmolol or propranolol will decrease the heart rate. When supraventricular or recurrent ventricular tachycardia occurs before separation, one must search diligently for causes. This may be a time to reassess the patient's chemical status. Cardioversion, overdrive pacing, or antiarrhythmic drugs may be necessary. Occasionally a left or right atrial catheter has slipped into the left or right ventricle, generating an artifactual irritable focus. The latter is often overlooked, yet is simple and productive of a dramatic "cure" when discovered.

ST segment elevation is a common finding immediately after restoration of cardiac rhythm before termination of bypass. In a study of patients undergoing coronary artery bypass grafting, Thomson et al.[18] found a 43 per cent incidence of ST segment elevation during emergence from bypass. The elevation may be due to ischemia from coronary embolism, coronary spasm or thrombosis, epicardial injury, temperature gradient, or inhomogeneous reperfusion, and, although these are pathologic, it is usually transient (i.e., over time ST segments return to baseline). When persistent elevation of ST segments suggests ischemia, more time on bypass and/or elevating mean arterial blood pressure may lead to improvement. If coronary artery spasm is suspected, intracoronary or intravenous nitroglycerin or intravenous calcium channel blockers may be indicated.[19, 20] Sublingual nifedipine has also been advocated, but this has not produced good results in our hands.

MONITORING DURING EMERGENCE FROM BYPASS

Before discontinuing bypass, all pressure transducers should be zeroed, their gains recalibrated; all monitoring catheters should be functioning properly with their distal ends in proper position. The position of the operating table should be checked. Is it level, or still in the head-down position for evacuation of air from the heart? Is it rotated to the left or right? Perhaps a slight head-down tilt is preferable during emergence because resumption of ventricular ejection may dislodge bubbles or emboli not previously removed, although there is no evidence one way or the other.

Radial arterial pressure may not reflect central aortic pressure,[21–23] a fact often noted at the end of CPB. The patient might thus appear severely hypotensive when in fact the central aortic pressure at least is satisfactory (Fig. 6–2). A cuff pressure is also a poor predictor of the aortic pressure. A pressure determination from a needle in the aorta can save administration of unnecessary inotropic drugs because low peripheral arterial pressures do not necessarily mean low central aortic blood pressure or low cardiac output (although this should be considered as a cause of the discrepancy).

DISCONTINUING BYPASS

At the time the patient is being separated from CPB, communication among anesthesiologists, surgeons, perfusionists, and nurses is critical.

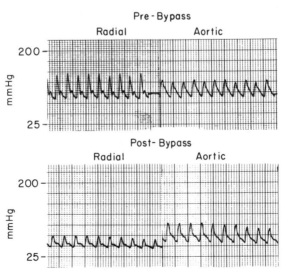

Figure 6–2. Photograph of data showing the reversal of usual relationships between simultaneous *aortic* and *radial* pressures after cardiopulmonary bypass in one patient. (From Stern DH, et al.: Can we trust the direct radial artery pressure immediately following cardiopulmonary bypass? Anesthesiology 62:558, 1985, with permission)

It is not a time for egos, or dogma, or insistence on "pet" therapies. As stated previously, it is a time when the anesthesiologist should have anticipated modalities that might be necessary to end bypass successfully. In the simplest form of separation from bypass, the venous line is occluded, and gradual replacement of the cardiac pressure and flow workload rapidly results in satisfactory hemodynamics. Before separation from bypass, the anesthesiologist should plan the fluids to be used after transfusion from the pump is complete. Will this be crystalloid, colloid, or blood products? Should these fluids be given through warmers? Also at this time the surgical field should be inspected for bleeding, integrity of suture lines, and, if caval tapes were used, that these have been fully released. Occasionally a vent will not have been removed. The need for inotropes or vasodilators should be thought about well in advance, especially if right or left ventricular failure is anticipated or was present before bypass. This is also a time to prepare any mechanical assist devices that might seem likely to be needed.

When should inotropic support and/or ventricular assist devices be anticipated (Table 6–2)? (1) A patient with evidence of severe preoperative ventricular dysfunction may need support after bypass. Abnormalities in exercise tolerance, persistent ischemia, recent infarction, ventricular failure, poor ejection fraction, increased left ventricular end diastolic pressure and wall motion are all clues but are by no means perfect predictors.[24] (2) The "quality" of myocardial preservation is another clue. Has the distribution of the cardioplegic solution been satisfactory? Has the heart remained cold with the proper maintenance schedule for readministration of cardioplegia, careful attention to topical hypothermia with ice, and protection from other sources of heat? The same considerations of myocardial preservation exist with intermittent cross-clamping techniques. (3) The "quality" of the surgical repair is important. Does the surgeon believe that the runoff distal to any coronary artery bypass grafts is good? Was a ventriculotomy necessary for the surgical procedure? (4) Length of cross-clamp time is important in anticipating immediate postoperative ventricular dysfunction. (5) Was the patient tolerant of depressant effects of anesthetics during induction and maintenance of anesthesia? If consideration of the above points toward likely need for inotropes, vasodilators, and/or mechanical assistance, these should be prepared and be ready to be instituted. By this it is meant that infusion

TABLE 6–2. ESTIMATION OF NEED FOR CIRCULATORY SUPPORT AFTER CARDIOPULMONARY BYPASS

1. Preoperative ventricular function
2. Circulatory response to anesthetics pre-bypass
3. Effectiveness of myocardial preservation
4. Quality of surgical repair
5. Aortic cross-clamp time

pumps should be ready and tested, and that initial dosages in micrograms per kilogram per minute has been translated into drops per minutes and routes of administration are agreed on. Scurrying in confusion to prepare inotropes while the heart struggles at high filling pressures should not occur.

As the surgeon (or perfusionist) occludes the venous line, blood volume is returned to the patient and cardiac workload is replaced. It has been stated that the length of time this process should take should be inversely related to anticipated postbypass myocardial function.[25] Filling the heart at this time is an exercise in the Starling mechanism. The patient is overtransfused (i.e., to the flat part of the Starling curve) when additional transfusion that increases left atrial and pulmonary artery diastolic pressure no longer results in additional elevation in arterial blood pressure. Often a left atrial or pulmonary artery occluded pressure of 10 to 15 mm Hg will be satisfactory. Those who use the transesophageal echo (TEE) would like to see the heart full but not distended, and are in a position to look for regional wall motion abnormalities, even to the point of being able to diagnose trouble with particular grafts. The TEE can also be used to check valve function—even to help make the decision whether or not to replace a valve (D. Thys, personal communication, 1988). Transfusion at the end of bypass should be individualized to achieve lowest ventricular filling pressures that generate adequate output. The ventricles, the atria, the pulmonary artery, and thermodilution outputs are gross indicators but are often unreliable during these first critical minutes. The arterial waveform may be of some help in assessing adequate filling volumes. Later, measurement of cardiac output and calculation of systemic vascular resistance will assist in the "fine tuning" of hemodynamics. *Overtransfusion with left ventricular distention must be avoided at all costs.* This can lead to poor subendocardial blood flow and decreased coronary perfusion pressure, and the resultant subendocardial ischemia may lead to even lower blood pressure with a vicious circle of problems. Also, mitral regurgitation can be produced, caused by mechanical distention and posterior papillary muscle ischemic dysfunction.

When ventricular filling pressures are mildly elevated and blood pressure is slightly low during initial separation from bypass, all that may be needed, if anything, is a small intravenous bolus of inotrope (e.g., ephedrine, 10 mg). This is many times sufficient to restore satisfactory blood pressure with a decrease in filling pressure to normal values. Another agent that has been used in this situation has been calcium chloride. Proponents of its use argue that calcium is a time-tested therapy for improving hemodynamics after bypass, that patients are often hypocalcemic at the end of bypass anyway, and that calcium will offset effects of the potassium cardioplegic solution. When calcium is administered intravenously, its hemodynamic effects can be expected to last for 10 to 20 minutes.[26-28] Controversy exists as to the effects of calcium on the myocardium and on the peripheral circulation, and as to the frequency of hypocalcemia that can be expected after bypass. In a study by Lappas et al.[29] 5 mg/kg of intravenous calcium chloride was administered immediately after bypass. Increases in blood pressure and systemic vascular resistance and decreased left ventricular filling pressure were noted. There were no important changes in heart rate or cardiac index. The question was asked whether the improvement in contractility was due to the calcium directly or because increased afterload, and the consonant increased inotropic state to overcome it, resulted in increased blood pressure and coronary flow. Auffant et al.[30] found hypocalcemia to be a frequent occurrence after bypass, but ionized calcium levels did not correlate well with hemodynamic state. Heining et al.[31] found no important changes in ionized calcium during bypass. They measured a wide range of ionized calcium levels immediately after bypass and concluded that the Ca^{++} level did not affect myocardial performance. Their paper recommends giving calcium for specific hemodynamic indications only, not just to increase the plasma ionized calcium level per se. A recent review by Drop reported a study wherein doses of 3 to 15 mg/kg of calcium chloride, given to adults, were actively followed by declines in serum ionized calcium concentrations over the next 3 to 15 minutes. Changes in left ventricular function were small with only 10 per cent to 20 per cent increases in performance. The author also noted that elevated calcium levels can increase vascular resistance in the peripheral, coronary, renal, and cerebral beds.[27] In contrast, some studies have shown decreased systemic vascular resistance.[27] Drop also remarked on the potential for sinus arrhythmia, bradycardia, AV dissociation, or junctional rhythm after calcium administration. A study in animals by Scheidegger et al.[32] found that changes in mean arterial blood pressure were related to systemic vascular resistance rather than to large flow changes. The same group also reported that when calcium chloride was used to correct measured hypocalcemia, increased mean arterial blood pressure was due to improvements in stroke volume. In contrast, when calcium chloride was added to normocalcemic animals, mean arterial pressure increased secondary to increases in systemic vascular resistance.[33] With regard to pediatric patients, hypocalcemia at the end of bypass has been noted as well.[34, 35]

Even if administration of calcium chloride can improve myocardial function at the end of bypass, its administration may worsen residual myocardial ischemia[36] and/or produce coronary artery spasm.[37] Most anesthesiologists today use calcium chloride for selected patients at the end of bypass rather than as a routinely administered drug, and avoid calcium altogether if there is a likelihood of persistent myocardial ischemia or reperfusion injury.

When a single bolus of an inotropic drug has been ineffective or obvious severe left ventricular dysfunction is present, it is prudent to first return the patient to CPB support. This avoids struggling along with elevated left atrial pressure, hypotension, low cardiac output, and shock. It also allows everyone to regroup and communicate. The team must look for causes for the poor myocardial performance. Is this right or left ventricular failure? Are there mechanical problems with the heart, air or clot in the coronary bypass grafts, undetected or unimproved gradients across cardiac valves, or is a ventricular septal defect present? Another important consideration in this situation is postischemic (i.e., post-cross-clamp) global myocardial dysfunction,[24, 38, 39] a relatively common problem.[24] Further increases in filling do not improve cardiac output and may worsen the situation by actually causing decreased ventricular ejection.[40] There is evidence that simply "resting" the heart on bypass may be beneficial.[41, 42] "Premature" use of inotropes has even been contended to be detrimental in one study.[43] Nonetheless, with the patient back on bypass and some control of the circulation, infusion of an inotropic drug can be started and the patient slowly weaned.

INOTROPIC AGENTS

The ideal inotropic drug would increase contractility and ventricular ejection without elevations in heart rate, systemic vascular resistance, or myocardial oxygen consumption. This agent does not exist. Instead, the anesthesiologist must estimate the status of the circulation and individualize the choice from one of the inotropic drugs currently available. The most common problem in adults is left ventricular dysfunction. In this situation, *epinephrine* will exert strong inotropic action without tachyphylaxis. As the infusion rate increases, increases in peripheral vascular resistance occur as increased alpha-adrenergic stimulation occurs. Epinephrine also causes venous constriction with consonant increased biventricular preload, and may reduce renal blood flow. The desired effects of epinephrine on the circulation may not be fully realized if the patient is acidotic, so concomitant alkalinization may help. Many experienced cardiovascular anesthesiologists rely on epinephrine because of its potency and versatility and because it is, indeed, the body's evolved substance for crisis states. It has always been the drug of first choice in traditional situations of cardiac arrest. Many experienced cardiovascular anesthesiologists agree that the end of CPB is not the time for trials at first with weaker drugs, risking continued myocardial failure when trying to separate the patient from bypass. These drug failures represent, inevitably, extra time spent at high filling and low coronary perfusion pressures. If an exogenous inotrope is indicated, *initially* using a strong inotropic agent (e.g., epinephrine) often allows relatively smooth separation from bypass on the first attempt, with reasonable ventricular filling pressures, blood pressure, and cardiac output. Increases in myocardial oxygen demand with epinephrine in the patient with coronary artery disease are much less of a concern after bypass because the major coronary lesions have been bypassed. Indeed, to *allow* the muscle to use more oxygen is a reasonable definition of positive inotropy. After successful discontinuation of CPB and achievement of satisfactory mean arterial blood pressure, attention can be directed to other circulatory issues. These include blood gas measurement, measurement of cardiac output and urine output, calculation of systemic vascular resistance, concomitant use of vasodilators, and the substitution and/or addition of other inotropic drugs. *It seems much more reasonable to start this "resuscitation" with the traditional advanced cardiac life support drug— epinephrine—and then taper to drugs that might be less harsh on the renal blood flow, rather than risk the several failures mentioned above.* If all that is "needed" *initially* to separate a patient from bypass is dopamine, we wonder if any exogenous inotrope was in fact needed.

High infusion rates of epinephrine may produce tachycardia or arrhythmias. Substitution of norepinephrine or addition of mechanical circulatory support may be necessary when such arrhythmias occur and/or desired systemic blood pressure cannot be achieved with epinephrine, especially when systemic resistance is persistently low. Other catecholamines—dopamine, dobutamine, isoproterenol, and norepinephrine—do have a place in emergence from bypass. Abnormalities in cardiac output, systemic vascular resistance, pulmonary vascular resistance, urine output, or biventricular function may be indications for initial use of one or more of these inotropes or a change to one of them.

Many studies have compared various inotropic drugs at the end of bypass.[44-58] Stephenson et al.[48] compared four infusion rates of dopamine with four infusion rates of epinephrine in postoperative cardiac patients several hours after termination of bypass. They found the hemodynamic effects of the drugs to be similar except for an increase in urine output with the use of dopamine.[48] Steen et al.[49] measured the hemodynamic effects of dopamine, dobutamine, or epinephrine during actual emergence from bypass in patients considered candidates for exogenous inotrope administration. All drugs increased cardiac index with a wide variance among these patients but with the greatest beta-induced systemic resistance decrease owing to dopamine, and unfortunately quite flat dose–response curves for both dopamine and dobutamine compared with epinephrine. This study and others[46, 47, 50-52] note improvements in hemodynamics with dopamine, dobutamine, or epinephrine without unwanted chronotropic arrhythmogenic and beta dilatory effects often seen with isoproterenol. Infusion rates of 5, 10, and 15 μg/kg/min of dopamine were studied by Merin et al.[53] in a group of patients after bypass. They found the largest gain in cardiac output with the 5 μg/kg/min dose, again indicating a relatively flat dose–response curve for this agent in this situation. Dobutamine, at infusion rates of 5 and 10 μg/kg/min, was compared with isoproterenol during emergence from bypass at 0.02 μg/kg/min in a study by Tinker et al.[54] They noted such increased heart rate and unwanted arrhythmias in the isoproterenol group as to discontinue the study, which required isoproterenol to be given in protocol manner, rather than by titration to heart rate. Dobutamine did not change heart rate, but increased cardiac index and mean arterial pressure. In a similar study Lewis et al.[55] also found a smaller effect on heart rate and systemic vascular resistance with dobutamine when compared with isoproterenol among cardiac patients studied the day after surgery. DiSesa et al.[56] found similar increases in heart rate with dobutamine and dopamine at infusion rates of 2.5 and 5.0 μg/kg/min in cardiac patients 18 to 24 hours postoperatively. Solomon et al.[57] compared dopamine and dobutamine in patients 6 hours after coronary artery bypass grafting. The circulatory effects of the two drugs were similar at low doses, but infusion rates of 5.0 to 7.5 μg/kg/min of dopamine tended to increase blood pressure and systemic vascular resistance without changing the cardiac index. This was thought to be due to the increasing alpha-adrenergic effect of dopamine, and was not seen with dobutamine. Another problem with dopamine is that it is partially dependent on indirectly stimulating the release of endogenous catecholamines for its effect.[58] Summarizing these studies, only a few (as noted above) were done during actual emergence. Most were done with stable patients after conclusion of bypass. They do not show superiority of dobutamine over dopamine with respect to tachycardia, but they do show dobutamine to be more cardioselective (i.e., less productive of beta-induced muscle bed dilation) than either isoproterenol or dopamine. Epinephrine has a steeper dose-response curve, and is associated with less tachycardia but more venoconstriction than dopamine, dobutamine, or isoproterenol. Norepinephrine, sometimes useful when resistance is very low, has not been as extensively studied but is advocated by several respected cardiovascular anesthesia authorities, often in combination with individualized alpha blockade using phentolamine.

Vasodilators

As has been suggested with other instances of heart failure, attention must be paid to derangement of the peripheral circulation.[59] Increases in systemic vascular resistance may be present from stimulation of various hormonal systems. Infusions of vasopressors can cause further increases in systemic vascular resistance. Concomitant use of vasodilators and inotropes is often necessary in both adults and children after bypass.[60–63] Another use of vasodilators is to treat systemic hypertension after bypass. Drugs such as sodium nitroprusside, nitroglycerin, and phentolamine have been used to decrease systemic vascular resistance, which in turn may result in increased cardiac index and improved myocardial function. Nitroprusside and especially nitroglycerin will cause venodilation and decreased ventricular filling pressures. When using vasodilators to decrease systemic vascular resistance, hoping to get increased cardiac index, the upper limit of the infusion rate is determined by the minimum acceptable level of systemic arterial blood pressure, with the caveat that cyanide toxicity must always be kept in mind with nitroprusside.

Sodium nitroprusside is a commonly used vasodilator immediately after termination of bypass.[64–67] It rapidly reduces systemic vascular resistance in dose-dependent manner with little tachyphylaxis. It has been reported to improve cardiac index concomitant treatment of hypertension after bypass. One must not forget the possibility of cyanide toxicity with nitroprusside (do not use more than 8 μg/kg/min), nor that it is also a venodilator. Preload augmentation may be needed with use of nitroprusside if the potential gain in cardiac index through reduction of systemic vascular resistance is offset by too great a decrease in left ventricular filling pressure.

Similarly, nitroglycerin has been used to offset the alpha-adrenergic effects of inotropes as well as to treat hypertension. An early report by Dunbar[68] described use of intravenous nitroglycerin with epinephrine to aid in discontinuing bypass. Nitroglycerin was used in an attempt to reduce impedance to left ventricular ejection and to decrease preload. Also reported were increased stroke volume, decreased chamber size, decreased left ventricular stroke work, and decreased myocardial oxygen consumption. Nitroglycerin may indirectly produce a favorable redistribution of coronary blood flow. It is easily controlled and reversible; and it is nontoxic, except that an overdose may produce too great a decrease in arterial pressure or in ventricular filling pressure. When used for treatment of postoperative hypertension, nitroglycerin has been found to reduce right and left ventricular filling pressures further than sodium nitroprusside.[69, 70] Despite the above, clinicians generally find that if the primary clinical objective is reduction in arterial pressure, then nitroprusside works better.

Right Ventricular Failure During Emergence from Bypass

The presence of right instead of or in addition to left ventricular failure requires different considerations when choosing vasodilators and ino-

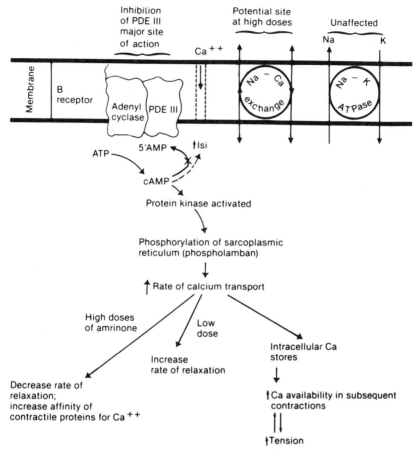

Figure 6-3. Postulated mechanism of action of amrinone. Ca = calcium; ↑ = increase; ↓ = decrease; ISi = slow inward calcium current; PDE = phosphodiesterase; X denotes inhibition. (From Mancini D, et al.: Intravenous use of amrinone for the treatment of the failing heart. Am J Cardiol 56:9B, 1985, with permission).

tropes. Right ventricular function, central venous pressure, pulmonary vascular resistance,[71–73] and ventilation, among other parameters, can become important. D'Ambra et al.[71] described use of prostaglandin E_1 for treatment of refractory heart failure and pulmonary hypertension after mitral valve replacement. Doses of prostaglandin E_1 (32–50 ng/kg/min) were infused into the right heart in combination with left atrial infusions of norepinephrine in five patients. This combination of drugs produced improvement in right ventricular function and allowed separation from bypass. Because isoproterenol is the only "pure" beta-adrenergic stimulator available, it is the only catecholamine that will not additionally constrict pulmonary vasculature. Right ventricular failure may, therefore, dictate a trial with isoproterenol. Some consider isoproterenol to be a pulmonary vasodilator. There is no evidence for this. If right ventricular output increases without much increased pulmonary artery pressure (i.e., without active pulmonary vasoconstriction), then pulmonary vascular resistance will have been decreased, not by active vasodilation, but merely by isoproterenol's lack of appreciable alpha activity. This may be of significant benefit if the right ventricle is failing, provided excessive tachycardia and dysrhythmias can be avoided.

Amrinone

Amrinone is a non-catecholamine, non-glycoside inotropic drug that has prominent vasodilating properties (Fig. 6–3). It may produce improvement in cardiac index, left ventricular end-diastolic pressure, systemic vascular resistance, and pulmonary vascular resistance, and usually does not change heart rate. Often it actually lowers blood pressure, whether this is desirable or not. Because of its effects on myocardial contractility and systemic vascular resistance, it behaves somewhat as a combination of inotrope and vasodilator. Its actions occur because it inhibits myocardial and vascular tissue phosphodiesterase, which leads to increased cyclic adenosine monophosphate. Its action seems limited to inhibition of only phosphodiesterase III. This proposed specificity of inhibition may account for its much greater effect on cardiac contractility than that of other phosphodiasterase inhibitors, which act nonspecifically on all forms of the enzyme. The effect on phosphodiesterase also accounts for the vasodilating action of amrinone. Amrinone is neither arrhythmogenic nor antiarrhythmic. An intravenous bolus of 0.75 mg/kg can be expected to produce an effect within 5 minutes[74] and is usually followed by an infusion of 2 to 10 μg/kg/min. Goenen et al.[75] have described use of amrinone for management of low cardiac output after cardiac surgery. In their study, amrinone was added to other inotropic drugs, vasodilators, and even the intra-aortic balloon pump to treat moderate and severe cardiac failure. Amrinone used in combination with other drugs markedly improved hemodynamic status by increasing cardiac index and decreasing ventricular filling pressures. A similar study by Gunnicker and Hess[76] investigated the effects of amrinone added to inotropic and vasodilator support for treatment of low cardiac output syndrome in 24 cardiac surgical patients after bypass. Amrinone increased cardiac index and blood pressure but decreased heart rate and systemic vascular resistance. This study did note an unwanted side effect—a marked decrease in platelets. Walker et al.[77] have reported that amrinone is reasonable for congestive heart failure in neonates.

MECHANICAL ASSIST DEVICES

Mechanical assist devices differ from pharmaceutical approaches in that they use external energy and do not require more work from the heart with concomitant increased myocardial oxygen consumption.[78-90] It may be necessary to use the intra-aortic balloon pump in addition to inotropes and vasodilators to wean the patient from bypass.[78, 79] As when considering the institution of inotropic drugs, one should never sit with a patient in shock, with a distended heart, low arterial pressures, developing acidosis, while pondering use of a mechanical assist device. The device must be inserted before this degree of deterioration, or the patient placed back on bypass during insertion. Taking this one step further, Feola et al.[80] described preoperative insertion of the intra-aortic balloon pump in patients with poor left ventricular function. The same considerations apply when the left or right ventricular assist device or the artificial heart is contemplated for use in separating the patient from the heart-lung machine, except that these patients may become candidates for cardiac transplantation. The anesthesiologist should not believe that early consideration of the balloon is a defeat or insult against his or her pharmacologic expertise. These devices do carry major risks, but do add hydraulic energy without requiring additional oxygen consumption.

SUMMARY

Emergence from bypass is a time of planning, organization, and cooperation among the cardiac operating room team. The cardiac anesthesiologist must prepare the patient for separation from bypass and correct metabolic or physiologic abnormalities that can be ameliorated. Monitoring equipment must be checked, and vasoactive drugs and mechanical assist devices anticipated and made ready, if thought necessary during careful pre-emergence planning. Early intervention with potent drugs and mechanical assist devices should be the rule. Periods of pharmacologic and mechanical support after bypass are better than periods of heart failure with high filling pressures and low output, with vital organ ischemia, while time is spent proving that weaker drugs are unsatisfactory. Initial therapy with epinephrine makes sense (i.e., taper to weaker inotropes later rather than the other way around). After successful weaning from bypass, attention can be directed to other important factors such as systemic vascular resistance, cardiac output, renal perfusion, and adequacy of gas exchange.

References

1. Lilly JK, Boland JP, Zekam S: Urinary bladder temperature monitoring: A new index of core body temperature. Crit Care Med 8:742–744, 1980.
2. Bone ME, Feneck RO: Bladder temperature as an estimate of body temperature during cardiopulmonary bypass. Anaesthesia 43:181–185, 1988.
3. Ramsay JG, Ralley FE, Whalley DG, et al: Site of temperature monitoring and prediction of afterdrop after open heart surgery. Can Anaesth Soc J 32:607–612, 1985.
4. Sladen RN: Temperature and ventilation after hypothermic cardiopulmonary bypass. Anesth Analg 64:816–820, 1985.
5. Noback CR, Tinker JH: Hypothermia after cardiopulmonary bypass in man. Anesthesiology 53:277–280, 1980.
6. Azar I: Rectal temperature is best indicator of adequate rewarming during cardiopulmonary bypass. Anesthesiology 55:189–190, 1981.
7. Muravchick S, Conrad DP, Vargas A: Peripheral temperature monitoring during cardiopulmonary bypass operation. Ann Thorac Surg 29:36–41, 1980.
8. Stanley TH, Jackson J: The influence of blood flow and arterial blood pressure during cardiopulmonary bypass on deltoid muscle gas tensions and body temperature after bypass. Can Anaesth Soc J 26:277–281, 1979.
9. Williams DG, Siefen AB, Lawson NW, et al: Pulsatile perfusion versus conventional high-flow nonpulsatile perfusion for rapid core cooling and rewarming of infants for circulatory arrest in cardiac operation. J Thorac Cardiovasc Surg 78:667–677, 1978.
10. Gravlee GP: Delayed rewarming during cardiopulmonary bypass. In Reves JG, Hall KD (eds): Common Problems in Cardiac Anesthesia. Chicago, Year Book, 1987, pp 66–74.
11. Ellis FR, Zwana SLV: Thermal balance during cardiopulmonary bypass with moderate hypothermia in man. Br J Anaesth 49:1127–1132, 1977.
12. Singh RKK, Barratt-Boyes BG, Harris EA: Does pulsatile flow improve perfusion during hypothermic cardiopulmonary bypass? J Thorac Cardiovasc Surg 79:822–832, 1980.
13. Caldwell C, Crawford R, Sinclair I: Hypothermia after cardiopulmonary bypass in man. Anesthesiology 55:86–87, 1981.
14. Ralley FE, Ramsay JG, Wynand JE, et al: Effect of heated humidified gases on temperature drop after cardiopulmonary bypass. Anesth Analg 63:1106–1110, 1984.
15. Price SL, Brown DL, Carpenter RL, et al: Isoflurane elimination via a bubble oxygenator during extracorporeal circulation. J Cardiothorac Anesth 2:41–44, 1988.
16. Gothard JWW, Branthwaite MA: Anesthesia for Cardiac Surgery and Allied Procedures. Boston, Blackwell Scientific, 1987, pp 120–122.
17. Lake CL, Sellers D, Nolan SP, et al: Energy dose and other variables possibly affecting ventricular defibrillation during cardiac surgery. Anesth Analg 63:743–751, 1984.
18. Thomson IR, Rosenbloom M, Cannon JE, Morris A: Electrocardiographic ST-segment elevation after myocardial reperfusion during coronary artery surgery. Anesth Analg 66:1183–1186, 1987.
19. Buxton AE, Goldberg S, Harken A, et al: Coronary artery spasm after myocardial revascularization: Recognition and management. N Engl J Med 304:1249–1253, 1981.
20. Nussmeier NA, Slogoff S: Verapamil treatment of intraoperative coronary artery spasm. Anesthesiology 62:539–541, 1985.
21. Stern DH, Gerson JI, Allen FB, Parker FB: Can we trust the direct radial artery pressure immediately following cardiopulmonary bypass? Anesthesiology 62:557–571, 1985.
22. Mohr R, Lavee J, Goor DA: Inaccuracy of radial artery pressure measurement after cardiac operations. J Thorac Cardiovasc Surg 94:286–290, 1987.
23. Gallagher JD, Moore RA, McNicholas KW, Joge AB: Comparison of radial and femoral arterial blood pressure in children after cardiopulmonary bypass. J Clin Monitor 1:168–171, 1985.
24. Mangano DT: Biventricular function after myocardial revascularization in human: Deterioration and recovery patterns after the first 24 hours. Anesthesiology 62:517–527, 1985.
25. Amado WJ, Starr NJ, Thomas SJ: Intraoperative management for open heart surgery. In

Thomas SJ (ed): Manual of Cardiac Anesthesia. New York, Churchill Livingstone, 1986, p 355.

26. Denlinger JK, Kaplan JA, Lecky JH, Wollman H: Cardiovascular responses to calcium administered intravenously to man during halothane anesthesia. Anesthesiology 42:390–397, 1985.

27. Drop LS: Ionized calcium, the heart and hemodynamic function. Anesth Analg 64:432–451, 1985.

28. Shapira N, Schaff HV, White RD, Pluth JR: Hemodynamic effects of calcium chloride injection following cardiopulmonary bypass. Ann Thorac Surg 37:133–140, 1984.

29. Lappas DG, Drop LJ, Buckley MJ, et al: Hemodynamic response to calcium chloride during coronary artery surgery. Surg Forum 26:234–235, 1975.

30. Auffant RA, Downs JB, Amick R: Ionized calcium concentration and cardiovascular function after cardiopulmonary bypass. Arch Surg 116:1072–1076, 1981.

31. Heining MPD, Linton RAF, Band DM: Plasma ionized calcium during open heart surgery. Anaesthesia 40:237–241, 1985.

32. Scheidegger D, Drop LJ, Schellenberg J-C: Role of the systemic vasculature in the hemodynamic response to changes in plasma ionized calcium. Arch Surg 115:206–211, 1980.

33. Drop LJ, Scheidegger D: Plasma ionized calcium concentration. J Thorac Cardiovasc Surg 79:425–431, 1980.

34. Abbott TR: Changes in serum calcium fractions and citrate concentrations during massive blood transfusions and cardiopulmonary bypass. Br J Anaesth 55:753–760, 1983.

35. Das JB, Eraklis AJ, Adams JG, Gross RE: Changes in serum ionic calcium during cardiopulmonary bypass with hemodilation. J Thorac Cardiovasc Surg 62:449–453, 1971.

36. Cheung JY, Bonventre JV, Molis CD, Leaf A: Calcium and ischemic injury. N Engl J Med 314:1670–1676, 1986.

37. Boulanger M, Maille JG, Pelletier GB, Michalk S: Vasopastic angina after calcium injection. Anesth Analg 63:1124–1126, 1984.

38. Tinker JH: Controversies about physiology and pharmacology during emergence from cardiopulmonary bypass. 1985 Review Course Lectures, International Anesthetic Research Society.

39. Braunwald E, Kloner RA: The stunned myocardium: Prolonged, post ischemic ventricular dysfunction. Circulation 66:1146–1149, 1982.

40. Mangano DT, Van Dyke DC, Ellis RJ: The effect of increasing preload on ventricular output and ejection in man. Circulation 62:535–541, 1980.

41. Levitsky S, Wright RW, Rao KS, et al: Does intermittent coronary perfusion offer greater myocardial protection than continuous aortic crossclamping? Surgery 82:51–59, 1977.

42. Tarhan S, White RD, Moffitt EA: Anesthesia and postoperative care for cardiac operations. Ann Thorac Surg 23:173–193, 1977.

43. Lazar HL, Buckberg GD, Foglia RP, et al: Detrimental effects of premature use of inotropic drugs to discontinue cardiopulmonary bypass. J Thorac Cardiovasc Surg 82:18–25, 1981.

44. Sakamoto T, Yamada T: Hemodynamic effects of dobutamine in patients following open heart surgery. Circulation 558:525–533, 1977.

45. Kersting F, Follath F, Moulds R, et al: A comparison of cardiovascular effects of dobutamine and isoprenaline after open heart surgery. Br Heart J 38:662–666, 1976.

46. d'Hollander A, Primo G, Hennart D, et al: Compared efficacy of dobutamine and dopamine in association with calcium chloride on termination of cardiopulmonary bypass. J Thorac Cardiovasc Surg 83:264–271, 1982.

47. Rosenblum R, Frieden J: Intravenous dopamine in the treatment of myocardial dysfunction after open heart surgery. Am Heart J 838:743–748, 1972.

48. Stephenson LW, Blackstone EH, Kouchoukos NT: Dopamine vs. epinephrine following cardiac surgery: Randomized study. Surg Forum 27:272–275, 1976.

49. Steen PA, Tinker JH, Pluth JR, et al: Efficacy of dopamine, dobutamine and epinephrine during emergence from cardiopulmonary bypass in man. Circulation 57:378–384, 1978.

50. Holloway EL, Stinson EB, Derby GC, Harrison DC: Action of drugs in patients early after cardiac surgery. Am J Cardiol 35:656–659, 1975.
51. Beregovich J, Reicher-Reiss H, Kunstadt D, Grishman A: Hemodynamic effects of isoproterenol in cardiac surgery. J Thorac Cardiovasc Surg 62:957–964, 1971.
52. Filner B, Karliner JS, Daily PO: Favorable influence of dopamine on left ventricular performance in patients refractory to discontinuation of cardiopulmonary bypass. Circ Shock 4:223–230, 1977.
53. Merin G, Bitran D, Uretzky G, et al: The hemodynamic effects of dopamine following cardiopulmonary bypass. Ann Thorac Surg 23:361–363, 1977.
54. Tinker JH, Tarhan S, White RD, et al: Dobutamine for inotropic support during emergence from cardiopulmonary bypass. Anesthesiology 44:281–286, 1976.
55. Lewis GRJ, Poole Wilson PA, Angerpointer TA, et al: Measurement of the circulatory effects of dobutamine, a new inotropic agent, in patients following cardiac surgery. Am Heart J 95:301–307, 1978.
56. DiSesa VJ, Brown E, Mudge GH, et al: Hemodynamic comparison of dopamine and dobutamine in the postoperative volume-loaded, pressure-loaded and normal ventricle. J Thorac Cardiovasc Surg 83:256–263, 1982.
57. Salomon NW, Plachetka JR, Copeland JG: Comparison of dopamine and dobutamine following coronary artery bypass grafting. Ann Thorac Surg 33:48–54, 1982.
58. Scallan MJH, Gothard JWW, Branthwaite MA: Inotropic agents. Br J Anaesth 51:649–658, 1979.
59. LeJemtel TH, Sonnenblick EH: Should the failing heart be stimulated? N Engl J Med 310:1384–1385, 1984.
60. Miller DC, Stinson EB, Oyer PE, et al: Postoperative enhancement of left ventricular performance by combined inotropic vasodilator therapy with preload control. Surgery 88:108–117, 1980.
61. Kirsh MM, Bove E, Detmer M, et al: The use of levarterenol and phentolamine in patients with low cardiac output following open heart surgery. Ann Thorac Surg 29:26–31, 1978.
62. Benzing G, Helmsworth JA, Schreiber JT, Kaplan S: Nitroprusside and epinephrine for treatment of low output in children after open-heart surgery. Ann Thorac Surg 27:523–528, 1978.
63. Appelbaum A, Blackstone EH, Kouchoukos NT, Kirklin JW: Afterload reduction and cardiac output in infants after intracardiac surgery. Am J Cardiol 39:445–451, 1977.
64. Tyden H, Johansson L, Nystrom SO, Westerholm CJ: Myocardial performance early after aortic-coronary bypass surgery and the influence of nitroprusside infusion. Acta Anesthes Scand 23:480–492, 1979.
65. Bixler TJ, Gardner TJ, Donahoo JS, et al: Improved myocardial performance in postoperative cardiac surgical patients with sodium nitroprusside. Ann Thorac Surg 25:444–448, 1978.
66. Lappas DG, Lowenstein E, Waller J, et al: Hemodynamic effects of nitroprusside infusion during coronary artery operation in man. Circulation 54:4–10, 1976.
67. Meretoja OA, Laaksonen VO: Hemodynamic effects of preload and sodium nitroprusside in patients subjected to coronary artery bypass. Circulation 58:815–825, 1978.
68. Dunbar RW: Vasodilator treatment of heart failure after cardiopulmonary bypass. Anesth Analg 54:842–847, 1975.
69. Stinson EB, Holloway EL, Derby GC, et al: Control of myocardial performance early after open heart operations by vasodilator treatment. J Thorac Cardiovasc Surg 73:523–530, 1977.
70. Kaplan JA, Finlayson DC, Woodward S: Vasodilator therapy after cardiac surgery: A review of the efficacy and toxicity of nitroglycerin and nitroprusside. Can Anaesth Soc J 27:254–259, 1980.
71. D'Ambra MN, LaRaia PJ, Philbin DM, et al: Prostaglandin E: A new therapy for refractory right heart failure and pulmonary hypertension after mitral valve replacement. J Thorac Cardiovasc Surg 89:567–572, 1985.
72. van den Dungen JJAM, Karliczek GH, Brenken U, et al: The effect of prostaglandin E_1 in patients undergoing clinical cardiopulmonary bypass. Ann Thorac Surg 35:406–414, 1983.

73. Hammond GL, Cronau LH, Whittaker D, Gilles CN: Fate of prostaglandins E_1 and A_1 in the human pulmonary circulation. Surgery 81:716–721, 1977.
74. Wilmhurst PT, Thompson DS, Jenkins BS, et al: Haemodynamic effects of intravenous amrinone in patients with impaired left ventricular function. Br Heart J 49:77–82, 1983.
75. Goenen M, Pedemonte O, Baele P, Col J: Amrinone in the management of low cardiac output after open heart surgery. Am J Cardiol 56:3B–38B, 1985.
76. Gunnicker M, Hess W: Preliminary results with amrinone in perioperative low cardiac output syndrome. J Thorac Cardiovasc Surg 35:219–225, 1987.
77. Walker PC, Perry BL, Shankaran S: Safety of amrinone for treating congestive heart failure in a premature neonate. Clin Pharmacol 6:326–331, 1987.
78. Sturm JT, Fuhrman TM, Sterling R, et al: Combined use of dopamine and nitroprusside therapy in conjunction with intra-aortic balloon pumping for the treatment of postcardiotomy low-output syndrome. J Thorac Cardiovasc Surg 82:1347, 1981.
79. Berger RL, Saini V, Ryan TJ, et al: Intra-aortic balloon assist for postcardiotomy cardiogenic shock. J Thorac Cardiovasc Surg 66:906–915, 1973.
80. Feola M, Weiner L, Walinsky P, et al: Improved survival artery coronary bypass surgery in patients with poor left ventricular function: Role of intraaortic balloon counterpulsation. Am J Cardiol 39:1021–1026, 1977.
81. Bregman D, Parodi EN, Haubert SM, et al: Counterpulsation with a new pulsatile assist device (PAD) in open-heart surgery. Med Instrument 10:232–238, 1976.
82. Tobias MA, Challen PD, Franklin CB, et al: Intra-aortic balloon counterpulsation. Anaesthesia 34:844–854, 1978.
83. Pennington DG, Swartz M, Codd JE, et al: Intraaortic balloon pumping in cardiac surgical patients: A nine-year experience. Ann Thorac Surg 36:125–131, 1983.
84. Subramanian VA, Goldstein JE, Sos TA, et al: Preliminary clinical experience with percutaneous intraaortic balloon pumping. Circulation 62:123–129, 1980.
85. Veasy LG, Blalock RC, Orth JL, Boucek MM: Intra-aortic balloon pumping in infants and children. Circulation 68:1095–1100, 1983.
86. Pierce WS, Parr GVS, Myers JL, et al: Ventricular-assist pumping in patients with cardiogenic shock after cardiac operation. N Engl J Med 305:1606–1610, 1981.
87. Kaplan JA, Craver JM, Jones EL, Sumpter R: The role of the intra-aortic balloon in cardiac anesthesia and surgery. Am Heart J 98:580–586, 1979.
88. Kopman EA, Ramierz-Inawat K: Intra-aortic balloon counterpulsation for right heart failure. Anesth Analg 59:74–76, 1980.
89. Balooki H, Williams W, Thurer RJ, et al: Clinical and hemodynamic criteria for use of the intra-aortic balloon pump in patients requiring cardiac surgery. J Thorac Cardiovasc Surg 72:756–768, 1976.
90. McGee MG, Zillgitt LG, Trono R, et al: Retrospective analysis of the need for mechanical circulatory support (Intraaortic balloon pump/abdominal left ventricular assist device or partial artificial heart) after cardiopulmonary bypass. Am J Cardiol 46:135–140, 1980.

CHAPTER 7

THE POSTPERFUSION SYNDROME: Inflammation and the Damaging Effects of Cardiopulmonary Bypass

JAMES K. KIRKLIN

THE CLINICAL SYNDROME

Most patients who undergo operations using cardiopulmonary bypass (CPB) as a support technique currently experience few identifiable adverse sequelae and convalesce normally. However, it is likely that all patients have a rather specific physiologic response that, in the occasional patient, will have markedly deleterious effects. In its severest form this adverse response to CPB has been termed the postperfusion syndrome, and may include, to a greater or lesser extent, clinical signs of pulmonary dysfunction, renal dysfunction, an abnormal bleeding diathesis, increased susceptibility to infection, increased interstitial fluid, leukocytosis, fever, vasoconstriction, and hemolysis.

The damaging effects of CPB probably relate to the abnormal events of bypass, including exposure to nonendothelial (unphysiologic) surfaces, shear stresses, and incorporation of abnormal substances during bypass (Fig. 7–1). This chapter focuses on those aspects of damage related to a generalized inflammatory response to the events of CPB.

THE HUMORAL AMPLIFICATION SYSTEMS

We and others have hypothesized that the damaging effects of CPB are related to the exposure of blood to various abnormal conditions, which then initiate a systemic "inflammatory response" involving both formed and unformed blood elements that normally act locally at sites of injury.

131

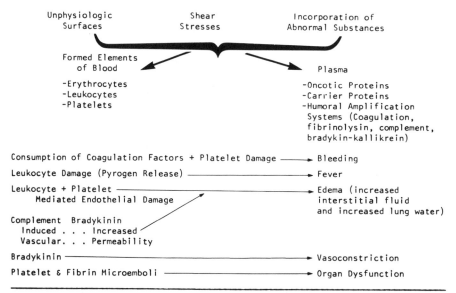

Figure 7–1. Schematic representation of the damaging effects of the exposure of blood to the abnormal events of cardiopulmonary bypass. (Reproduced with permission from Kirklin JK: Cardiopulmonary bypass. *In* Arciniegas E (ed): Pediatric Cardiac Surgery. Chicago, Year Book Medical Publishers, Inc., 1985, p 70.)

An integral part of this "whole body inflammatory response" involves the so-called humoral amplification system. This includes the coagulation cascade, the kallikrein cascade, the fibrinolytic system, and the complement system. The coagulation cascade is activated almost immediately after onset of CPB by exposure of blood to nonendothelial surfaces.[1, 2] Activation of Hageman factor (XII), and undoubtedly other events and substances, leads to activation of the kallikrein system and production of bradykinin. Bradykinin produces alterations in vascular permeability, initiates smooth muscle contraction, and dilates precapillary arterioles. High circulating bradykinin levels have been documented during CPB,[3, 4] particularly in infants.[5] Activation of the fibrinolytic system is also initiated at the onset of CPB,[6] and plasmin (the active fibrinolytic agent) may further activate prekallikrein, the complement system, and Hageman factor.

COMPLEMENT AND CARDIOPULMONARY BYPASS

The complement system comprises a group of circulating glycoproteins and forms the basic matrix of the body's response to immunologic injury, infections, or traumatic insult. Two pathways exist for complement activation (Fig. 7–2).[7] The classic pathway is usually initiated by means

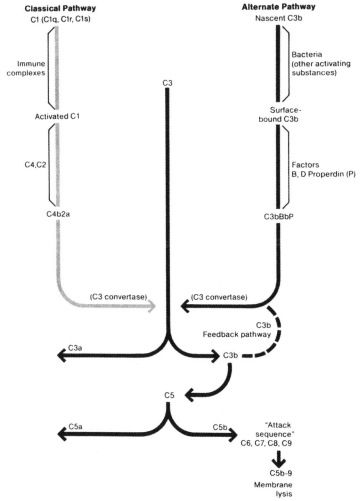

Figure 7-2. Pathways of complement activation. (Reproduced with permission from Goldstein IM: Current Concepts: Complement in Infectious Diseases. Kalamazoo, Michigan, The Upjohn Company, 1980, p 7.)

of interaction with antigen-antibody complexes, whereas the alternative, or properdin, pathway is generally activated by exposure of blood to foreign surfaces.[8]

Although earlier studies[9] had demonstrated complement consumption during CPB and even hypothesized a relation between complement activation and increased capillary permeability after CPB, Chenoweth et al.[8] at the University of Alabama at Birmingham and Scripps Institute first demonstrated in 1981 that complement anaphylatoxin C3a is released shortly after onset of CPB, with continued production throughout the duration of bypass (Fig. 7–3). Although some controversy exists, it is generally acknowledged that complement is activated predominantly by means of the alternative (properdin) pathway at the onset of CPB.[10]

Although complement activation has been demonstrated during operative procedures without CPB, the magnitude of activation is small compared with activation during CPB. In cardiac operations without CPB, for example, levels of C3a are essentially normal at the completion of the procedure (Fig. 7–4).[11] Fosse et al.[12] have also demonstrated increased levels of the terminal complement complex (TCC) shortly after the initiation of CPB (Fig. 7–5). TCC represents the end product of complement activation, and requires splitting of C5 into C5a and C5b.[12] In contrast, patients undergoing thoracotomy without CPB showed no increase in TCC levels (Fig. 7–6).[12]

A prospective clinical study at the University of Alabama examined variables related to CPB and their relation to morbidity after cardiac surgery.[11] Cardiac dysfunction (first 24 hours) after cardiac surgery was significantly related to higher C3a levels three hours after CPB, longer duration of CPB, and younger age at operation (Table 7–1). Similarly, postoperative pulmonary dysfunction was related to the same risk factors (Table 7–2). Risk factors specific for postoperative renal dysfunction included higher C3a levels 3 hours after CPB and younger age (Table 7–3). An overall index of morbidity was also determined that related significantly to higher levels of C3a, longer duration of CPB, and younger age at operation (Fig. 7–7). This relation between morbidity after CPB and complement activation is particularly interesting, since the anaphylatoxins C5a and C3a have physiologic effects similar to those observed

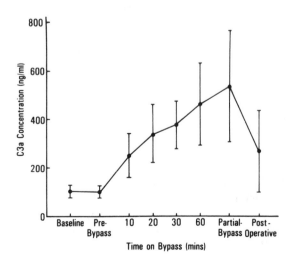

Figure 7–3. Plasma levels of C3a in patients undergoing cardiopulmonary bypass. (Reproduced with permission from Chenoweth et al: Complement activation during cardiopulmonary bypass: Evidence for generation of C3a and C5a anaphylatoxins. N Engl J Med 304:497, 1981.)

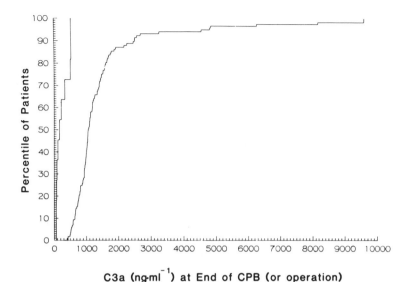

C3a (ng·ml⁻¹) at End of CPB (or operation)

Figure 7–4. C3a levels (ng·ml⁻¹) at the end of cardiopulmonary bypass, expressed in a cumulative percentile plot. The steep vertical line on the left represents closed heart patients, 100 per cent of whom had near-normal or normal levels. The curve on the right represents open heart patients, virtually all of whom had increased levels. Fifty per cent had levels above 1,000 (ng·ml⁻¹) and 25 per cent had levels above 1,600. (Reproduced with permission from Kirklin JK et al: Complement and the damaging effects of cardiopulmonary bypass. J Thorac Cardiovasc Surg 86:845, 1983.)

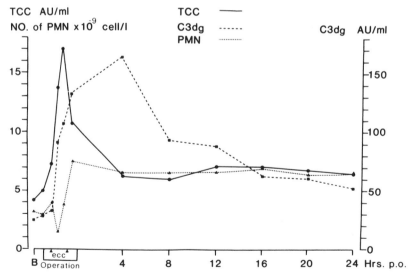

Figure 7–5. The concentration of TCC, C3dg, and PMNs in blood in ten patients undergoing aorta-coronary bypass operations during extracorporeal circulation (ecc) (median values). PMN, polymorphonuclear neutrophils. (Reproduced with permission from Fosse et al: Complement activation during major operations without cardiopulmonary bypass. J Thorac Cardiovasc Surg 93:860–866, 1987.)

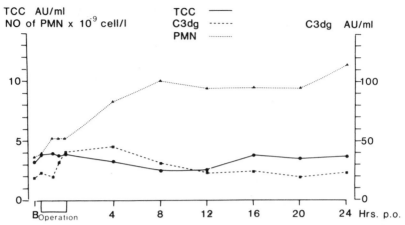

Figure 7–6. The concentration of TCC, C3dg, and PMNs in blood in five patients undergoing thoracotomy (median values). (Reproduced with permission from Fosse et al: Complement activation during major operations without cardiopulmonary bypass. J Thorac Cardiovasc Surg 93:860–866, 1987.)

in many patients after CPB, including vasoconstriction and increased capillary permeability.[13]

ALTERATIONS IN MICROVASCULAR PERMEABILITY

Accumulation of extravascular fluid has often been described after CPB, with clinical manifestations that include increased pulmonary interstitial fluid without elevation of left atrial pressure, increased tissue and peripheral edema, and ascites. In 1966 Cleland et al.[14] at the Mayo Clinic noted progressive increases in extravascular fluid after cardiac operations that were directly related to the duration of CPB (Fig. 7–8). Despite this and many other studies documenting alterations in the distribution of fluid after CPB, direct evidence for alterations in capillary permeability was lacking. In 1987 Smith et al.[15] from Alabama provided the first direct evidence for increased microvascular permeability after CPB. Using ultrafiltration techniques in a dog model, a segment of small intestine was isolated, its lymphatic drainage cannulated, and the segment's venous pressure progressively increased over a 3-hour period to augment lymphatic flow. The colloid osmotic sieving ratio is determined by the minimum lymph–plasma protein concentration and was used as a measure of microvascular permeability.[16] The permeability to each of six sizes of plasma proteins measured by density gradient gel electrophoresis was determined. A systematic increase in permeability to proteins by two hours of normothermic CPB was demonstrated (Fig. 7–9), with larger molecules proportionately more affected (Fig. 7–10).

TABLE 7–1. CARDIAC DYSFUNCTION AFTER OPEN OPERATIONS*

Incremental Risk Factor	Logistic Coefficient ±SD	p Value
Higher C3a level	0.0010 ± 0.00042	0.02
Longer CP8 time	0.014 ± 0.0058	0.02
Younger age	−0.06 ± 0.138	≤0.0001
Intercepts: Grade> 1 = − 2.3 ± 0.71		
Grade> 2 = − 4.1 ± 0.82		

n = 116; 27 patients had events
SD = Standard deviation; CPB = cardiopulmonary bypass

TABLE 7–2. PULMONARY DYSFUNCTION AFTER OPEN OPERATIONS*

Incremental Risk Factor	Logistic Coefficient ±SD	p Value
Higher C3a level	0.0025 ± 0.00094	0.008
Longer CP8 time	0.025 ± 0.0111	0.02
Younger age	−1.17 ± 0.183	<0.0001
Intercepts: Grade> 1 = 0.5 ± 1.01		
Grade> 2 = 3.7 ± 1.12		

n = 116; 41 patients had events
SD = Standard deviation; CPB = cardiopulmonary bypass

TABLE 7–3. RENAL DYSFUNCTION AFTER OPEN OPERATIONS*

Incremental Risk Factor	Logistic Coefficient ±SD	p Value
Higher C3 level	0.0009 ± 0.00036	0.02
Younger age	−0.07 ± 0.142	≤0.0001
Intercepts: Grade> 1 = 10.5 ± 0.47		
Grade> 2 = − 0.9 ± 0.47		
Grade> 3 = − 1.6 ± 0.50		
Grade 4 = − 2.6 ± 0.60		

n = 116; 24 patients had events
SD = Standard deviation; CPB = cardiopulmonary bypass

*These three tables are used with permission from Kirklin JK, Westaby S, Blackstone EH, et al: Complement and the damaging effects of cardiopulmonary bypass. J Thorac Cardiovasc Surg 86:845, 1983.

COMPLEMENT AND PULMONARY DYSFUNCTION AFTER CARDIOPULMONARY BYPASS

Particularly in infants, pulmonary dysfunction associated with radiographic evidence of increased pulmonary interstitial fluid is a common accompaniment of CPB. Polymorphonuclear leukocytes have specific binding sites for the anaphylatoxin C5a generated during CPB.[17] In addition, transpulmonary sequestration of leukocytes has been demon-

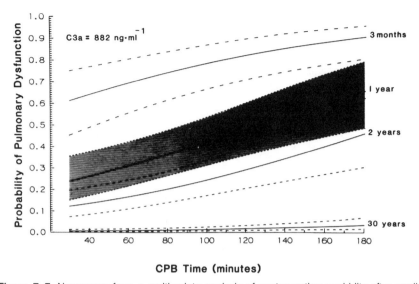

Figure 7–7. Nomogram from a multivariate analysis of postoperative morbidity after cardiac surgery. The significant risk factors included C3a level, age at operation, and duration of CPB. The shaded areas indicate the 70 per cent confidence limits for 60 minutes of CPB. (Reproduced with permission from Kirklin JK et al: Complement and the damaging effects of cardiopulmonary bypass. J Thorac Cardiovasc Surg 86:845, 1983.)

strated during partial bypass.[8] Flick et al.[18] demonstrated, using a sheep model with nitrogen mustard–induced leukopenia, that leukocytes were required for the increased pulmonary microvascular permeability that develops after microembolization. In the setting of hemodialysis, Craddock et al.[20] have demonstrated complement activation and related it to transient neutropenia and temporary pulmonary dysfunction.[19, 20]

More recently Salama et al.[21] from West Germany have also demonstrated deposition of the terminal C5b-9 complement complexes on erythrocytes and neutrophils during CPB. Intravascular hemolysis was observed in all patients, and C5b-9 was demonstrated on red cell ghosts but not on intact erythrocytes, inferring a relation between complement activation on red cells and hemolysis during CPB. In addition, granulocytes were found to nearly uniformly carry C5b-9 complexes during CPB and transiently afterward (less than 24 hours).

Based on these and other experimental studies and clinical observations, a current hypothesis for at least part of the pulmonary dysfunction seen after CPB would include the following: complement activation by way of the alternative (properdin) pathway leads to release of the anaphylatoxins C3a and C5a. C5a is rapidly bound to circulating neutrophils, which are then activated and undergo deposition and sequestration in the lungs as well as in other organs. The activated white cells release superoxides and lysosomal enzymes that then contribute to endothelial

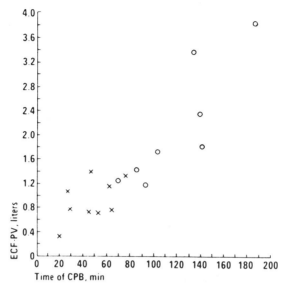

Figure 7–8. Relation between time of CPB and increment in extracellular fluid minus plasma volume (ECF-PV) soon after operation (post minus preoperative levels). x, open operation for L to R shunt; o, open operation for valvular heart disease (no congestive heart failure). (Reproduced from Cleland et al: Blood, volume and body fluid compartment changes soon after closed and open intracardiac surgery. J Thorac Cardiovasc Surg 52:698–705, 1966.)

injury, alterations in permeability, and accumulation of extravascular fluid.

PROTAMINE–COMPLEMENT INTERACTION

The deleterious response to CPB may be further complicated by accompanying pharmacologic interventions. This is particularly true with protamine sulfate, which is routinely used to reverse the anticoagulation effect of heparin after CPB. The anaphylatoxins C3a and C5a are generated by activation of either or both the classic and alternative pathways. In contrast, the anaphylatoxin C4a is generated only by activation of the classic pathway. In vitro studies demonstrated that human serum containing heparin alone or protamine sulfate alone does not activate complement, but the mixture of protamine sulfate and heparin in human serum results in marked activation of the classic pathway, with generation of C4a, C3a, and C5a (Fig. 7–11).[10] In a clinical study after coronary artery bypass surgery, we found elevated C3a and nearly normal C4a levels at the end of CPB. With administration of protamine sulfate, marked elevation of both C3a and C4a occurred, indicating activation of the classic complement pathway (Fig. 7–12).[10] Although unproved, it is

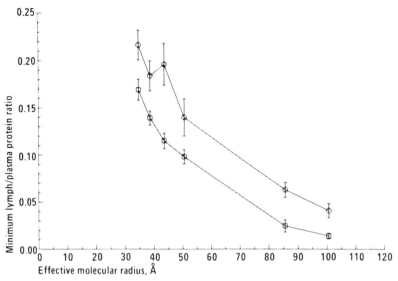

Figure 7–9. Relation of small intestinal microvascular colloid osmotic sieving ratio, as reflected by the minimum lymph-plasma protein ratio, to molecular radius in dogs undergoing either 2 hours of nonpulsatile normothermic CPB (o) or simple hemodilution with sham CPB (□). Shown are means + 1 SE for each group of seven dogs (p <.0001). (Reproduced with permission from Smith et al: Microvascular permeability after cardiopulmonary bypass. J Thorac Cardiovasc Surg 94:225–233, 1987.)

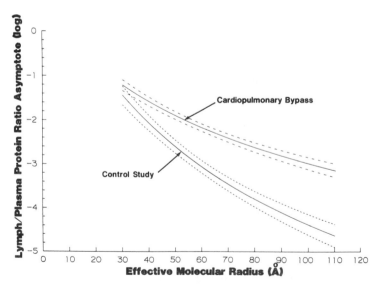

Figure 7–10. Nomogram relating the asymptote of the lymph-plasma protein ratio (permeability ratio) to the effective molecular radius of the proteins and to the conditions of the experiments (CPB or sham procedure). The vertical axis is in logarithmic units. (Reproduced with permission from Smith et al: Microvascular permeability after cardiopulmonary bypass. J Thorac Cardiovasc Surg 94:225–233, 1987.)

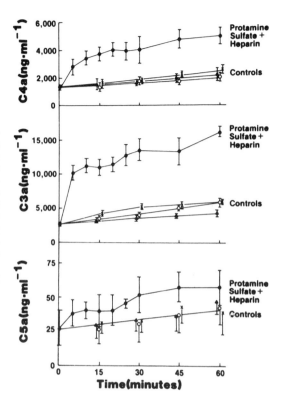

Figure 7–11. Levels of C4a, C3a, C5a in normal human serum incubated with a mixture of protamine sulfate and heparin (●). The controls consisted of human serum alone (▲), serum containing heparin (o), or serum containing protamine sulfate (x). (Reproduced with permission from The Society of Thoracic Surgeons. From Kirklin et al: Effects of protamine administration after cardiopulmonary bypass on complement, blood elements, and the hemodynamic state. Ann Thorac Surg 41:193–199, 1986.)

speculated that a more pronounced response to the protamine sulfate–heparin-induced activation of the classic complement activation pathway could induce some or all of the severe hemodynamic derangement that can occur after protamine administration.

REDUCTION OF THE INFLAMMATORY RESPONSE DURING CARDIOPULMONARY BYPASS

Although in this chapter we have related at least some of the damaging effects of CPB to a diffuse inflammatory response related in part to complement activation secondary to exposure of blood to nonendothelial surfaces of the pump oxygenator and bypass circuits, we do not as yet have secure proof of this hypothesis. It has, for example, been a widely appreciated clinical observation that the postperfusion syndrome is more rapidly ameliorated in the presence of robust cardiac performance and vice versa. This raises two possibilities: (1) that the same inflammatory responses attributed to CPB could be initiated within the body during,

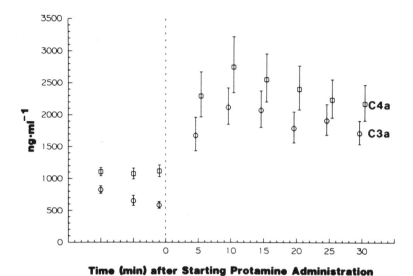

Figure 7–12. Levels of C3a and C4a after cardiopulmonary bypass (CPB) and the beginning of protamine sulfate administration × 0 and the broken vertical line indicate the beginning of protamine administration, which was 10 minutes after discontinuation of CPB. Protamine was infused over a 5-minute period. The vertical bars represent the 70 per cent confidence limits. The mean normal value of C3a is 76 ng·ml⁻¹ and for C4a, 1,200 ng·ml⁻¹. (Reproduced with permission from The Society of Thoracic Surgeons. From Kirklin et al: Effects of protamine administration after cardiopulmonary bypass on complement, blood elements, and the hemodynamic state. Ann Thorac Surg 41:193–199, 1986.)

or in some patients after, CPB by widespread micro areas of ischemia with or without necrosis; or (2) that robust cardiac performance somehow clears activated deleterious factors more effectively. Nonetheless, we do believe that promotion of robust cardiac performance early after operation, particularly with respect to our use of meticulous methods of myocardial protection and controlled reperfusion during and after global ischemia, may importantly reduce or shorten the duration of these damaging effects of CPB.

Many studies have also suggested that postbypass organ perfusion may be improved by certain technical aspects of the conduct of CPB. Hypothermia not only reduces cellular metabolic activity,[22–25] but also results in increased red cell aggregation and blood viscosity.[26] The latter may be counteracted by the beneficial effects of moderate hemodilution to improve cerebral, cardiac, and renal blood flows during bypass.[27] Whether there are real clinical benefits to the use of pulsatile flow during CPB with respect to organ perfusion remains controversial, and conflicting data exist regarding its potential benefit on lactate production and whole body oxygen consumption.[28–32]

There is no convincing evidence that the *type of oxygenator* used

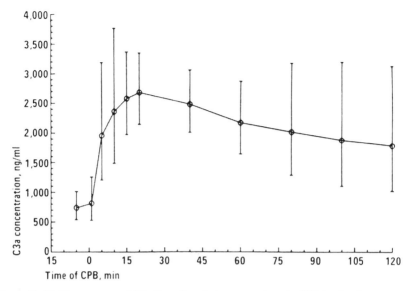

Figure 7–13. Time course of C3a liberation during normothermic CPB in pigs (mean + 1Sd). (Reproduced by permission of S. Karger AG, Basel, from Kirklin et al: Cardiopulmonary bypass: Studies on its damaging effects. Blood Purif 5:168–178, 1987.)

affects the magnitude of the inflammatory response. Using a radioim-munoassay for porcine C3a developed by Dr. Dennis Chenoweth, we have documented that there is similar response to CPB in the pig (i.e., with prompt and sustained elevation of C3a levels) as compared with man (Fig. 7–13).[33] In the pig model similar and marked complement activation with elaboration of C3a was observed with both a membrane oxygenator system and a bubble oxygenator system, the latter using either nylon or polypropylene mesh.

A clinical study reported by Cavarocchi et al.,[34] however, indicated a potentially favorable effect of a membrane oxygenator. A small but significant increment of C3a generation was noted with the bubble oxygenator at the end of CPB. This difference was accentuated with the administration of protamine (Fig. 7–14). The greater elaboration of C3a was accompanied by a significant increase in transpulmonary leukocyte sequestration at the end of bypass (Fig. 7–15). The administration of methylprednisolone (30 mg/kg) 20 minutes before CPB in the bubble oxygenator group eliminated any difference from the membrane oxyge-nator group in regard to both C3a elaboration and transpulmonary leukocyte sequestration (Figs. 7–14 and 7–15).[34]

In summary, CPB is known to activate the alternative (properdin) pathway of complement activation, and the magnitude of this activation is related to morbidity after cardiac surgery. Other damaging effects of CPB undoubtedly relate to an interaction between the other components

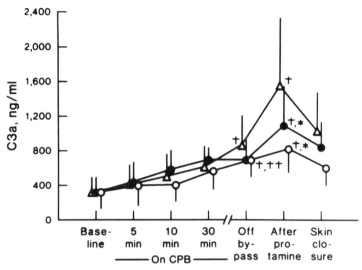

Figure 7-14. Plasma levels of C3a in patients undergoing cardiopulmonary bypass. Compared with the bubble oxygenator group (△), C3a levels in the bubble oxygenator group with Solu-Medrol (●) and the membrane oxygenator group (o) were significantly lower after bypass. Each point represents means ± SD. †, p <.0001 versus baseline; ‡, p <.02 versus bubble oxygenator group; *, p <.0001 versus bubble oxygenator group. (Reproduced with permission from Cavarocchi et al: Complement activation during cardiopulmonary bypass. J Thorac Cardiovasc Surg 91:252–258, 1986.)

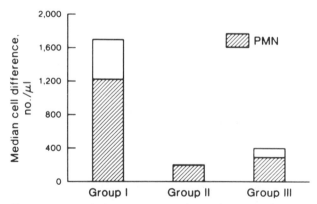

Figure 7-15. Transpulmonary leukocyte sequestration and neutropenia occurred after establishment of pulmonary circulation at conclusion of CPB. Transpulmonary leukocyte sequestration is expressed as median cell difference (MCD = WBC in right atrium—WBC in left atrium). Group 1, bubble oxygenator group; Group 2, bubble oxygenator group with Solu-Medrol; Group 3, membrane oxygenator group. (Reproduced with permission from Cavarocchi et al: Complement activation during cardiopulmonary bypass. J Thorac Cardiovasc Surg 91:252–258, 1986.)

of the humoral amplification system. Other blood components, such as activated platelets, further contribute organ damage or dysfunction. To date, specific refinements in the conduct of CPB designed to reduce the associated inflammatory response have been rather indirect. Whether specific blocking agents at critical steps of the complement cascade or the humoral amplification system would reduce these damaging effects is currently unknown and requires further investigation.

References

1. Feijen J: Thrombogenesis caused by blood foreign surface interaction. In Kenedit RM, Courtney JM, Gaylor JDS, Gilchrist T (eds): Artificial Organs. Baltimore, University Park Press, 1977, pp 235–247.
2. Verska JJ: Control of heparinization by activated clotting time during bypass with improved postoperative hemostasis. Ann Thorac Surg 24:170, 1977.
3. Ellison N, Behar M, MacVaugh H III, Marshall BE: Bradykinin, plasma protein fraction and hypotension. Ann Thorac Surg 29:15, 1980.
4. Pang LM, Stalcup SA, Lipset JS, et al: Increased circulating bradykinin during hypothermia and cardiopulmonary bypass in children. Circulation 60:1503, 1979.
5. Friedli B, Kent G, Olley PM: Inactivation of bradykinin in the pulmonary vascular bed of newborn and fetal lambs. Circ Res 33:421, 1973.
6. Backmann F, McKenna R, Cole ER, Najafi H: The hemostatic mechanism after open-heart surgery. I. Studies on plasma coagulation factors and fibrinolysis in 512 patients after extracorporeal circulation. J Thorac Cardiovasc Surg 70:76, 1975.
7. Goldstein IM: Current Concepts: Complement in Infectious Diseases. Upjohn Co, 1980, p 7.
8. Chenoweth DE, Cooper SW, Hugli TE, et al: Complement activation during cardiopulmonary bypass: Evidence for generation of C3a and C5a anaphylatoxins. N Engl J Med 304:497, 1981.
9. Parker DJ, Cantrell JW, Karp RB, et al: Changes in serum complement and immunoglobulins following cardiopulmonary bypass. Surgery 71:824, 1972.
10. Kirklin JK, Chenoweth DE, Naftel DC, et al: Effects of protamine administration after cardiopulmonary bypass on complement, blood elements, and the hemodynamic state. Ann Thorac Surg 41:193–199, 1986.
11. Kirklin JK, Westaby S, Blackstone EH, et al: Complement and the damaging effects of cardiopulmonary bypass. J Thorac Cardiovasc Surg 86:845, 1983.
12. Fosse E, Mollnes TE, Ingvaldsen B: Complement activation during major operations without cardiopulmonary bypass. J Thorac Cardiovasc Surg 93:860–866, 1987.
13. Muller-Eberhard HJ: Complement. Am Rev Biochem 44:697–724, 1975.
14. Cleland J, Pluth JR, Tauxe WN, Kirklin JW: Blood, volume and body fluid compartment changes soon after closed and open intracardiac surgery. J Thorac Cardiovasc Surg 52:698–705, 1966.
15. Smith EEJ, Naftel DC, Blackstone EH, Kirklin JW: Microvascular permeability after cardiopulmonary bypass. J Thorac Cardiovasc Surg 94:225–233, 1987.
16. Granger DN, Taylor AE: Permeability of intestinal capillaries to endogenous macromolecules. Am J Physiol 238:H457–464, 1980.
17. Chenoweth DE, Hugle TE: Demonstration of specific C5a receptor on intact human polymorphonuclear leukoctyes. Proc Natl Acad Sci USA 75:3943, 1978.
18. Flick MR, Perel A, Staub NC: Leukocytes are required for increased lung microvascular permeability after microembolization in sheep. Circ Res 48:344, 1981.
19. Craddock PR, Fehr J, Dalmasso AP, et al: Pulmonary vascular leukostasis resulting from complement activation by dialyzer cellophane membranes. J Clin Invest 59:879, 1977.

20. Craddock PR, Fehr J, Brigham KL, et al: Complement and leukocyte-mediated pulmonary dysfunction in hemodialysis. N Engl J Med 296:769, 1977.
21. Salama A, Hugo F, Heinrich D, et al: Deposition of terminal C5b-9 complement complexes on erythrocytes and leukocytes during cardiopulmonary bypass. J Thorac Cardiovasc Surg 88:101–112, 1985.
22. Fuhrman GJ, Fuhrman FA: Oxygen consumption of animals and tissues as a function of temperature. J Gen Physiol 42:715, 1959.
23. Penrod KE: Oxygen consumption and cooling rates in immersion hypothermia in the dog. Am J Physiol 157:436, 1949.
24. Shragge BW, Digerness SB, Blackstone EH: Complete recovery of the heart following exposure to profound hypothermia. J Thorac Cardiovasc Surg 81:455–458, 1981.
25. Treasure T, Naftel DC, Conger KA, et al: The effect of hypothermic circulatory arrest time on cerebral function morphology, and biochemistry. J Thorac Cardiovasc Surg 88:101–112, 1985.
26. Eiseman B, Spencer FC: Effect of hypothermia on the flow characteristics of blood. Surgery 52:532, 1961.
27. Utley JR, Wachtel C, Cain RB, et al: Effects of hypothermia, hemodilution, and pump oxygenation on organ water content, blood flow and oxygen delivery, and renal function. Ann Thorac Surg 31:121, 1981.
28. Trinkle JK, Helton NE, Wood RE, et al: Metabolic comparison of a new pulsatile pump and a roller pump for cardiopulmonary bypass. J Thorac Cardiovasc Surg 58:562, 1969.
29. Boucher JK, Rudy LW Jr, Edmunds H Jr: Organ blood flow during pulsatile cardiopulmonary bypass. J Appl Physiol 36:86, 1974.
30. Harken AH: The influence of pulsatile perfusion on oxygen uptake by the isolated canine hind limb. J Thorac Cardiovasc Surg 70:237, 1975.
31. Dunn J, Kirsh MM, Harness J, et al: Hemodynamic, metabolic, and hematologic effects of pulsatile cardiopulmonary bypass. J Thorac Cardiovasc Surg 84:1131–1135, 1981.
32. Shepard RB, Kirklin JW: Relation of pulsatile flow to oxygen consumption and other variables during cardiopulmonary bypass. J Thorac Cardiovasc Surg 58:694–702, 718–720, 1969.
33. Kirklin JK, Blackstone EH, Kirklin JW: Cardiopulmonary bypass: Studies on its damaging effects. Blood Purif 5:168–178, 1987.
34. Cavarocchi NC, Pluth JR, Schaff HV, et al: Complement activation during cardiopulmonary bypass. J Thorac Cardiovasc Surg 91:252–258, 1986.

INDEX

Note: Page numbers in *italics* refer to illustrations; page numbers followed by t refer to tables.

Acid-base management for hypothermic CPB, alpha-stat. See *Alpha-stat acid-base management.*
blood gas scale for, 1–2
CBF and CMRO$_2$ and, 24, 24–27, 35
comparison of strategies in, 1–2, 16t
correlation of CPB and MAP in, 25–27, 26
critical effects of, 2
early animal studies on, 3–4, 4
normal value adjustments for hypothermic patients, 2–3
organ function and preservation, 12–17
of brain, 12–14
of heart, 14–17
pH-stat. See *pH-stat acid-base management.*
theoretical implications for humans, 12
Acidosis, CPB emergence and, 119–120
during ischemia, 14–15
in hibernating mammals, 10
in hypothermia, brain function and, 14
Activated coagulation time (ACT), heparin anticoagulation neutralization and, 101–102
Adenosine monophosphate, cyclic, amrinone inhibition of, 124
Adenosine triphosphate (ATP), intracellular concentrations during ischemia, 14
perfusion flow rate and, 30–31
Adrenergic response, stress response and, 80
"Afterdrop" in temperature, during CPB emergence, 110–111
Age, and cerebral dysfunction, post-operative, 57
neuropsychologic dysfunction post-bypass and, 33, 48
prostaglandin metabolism during CPB, 84–85
stress response and, 80–81
stroke incidence post-bypass and, 47

Aggregation, cerebral autoregulation and, 14
embolism formation from, 34, 52
postperfusion syndrome and, 142
Air embolism. See *Macroembolism.*
Alcuronium, pharmacokinetics of, 74
Alfentanil, pharmacokinetics of, 74–75
stress response and, 88
Alkaline pH-stat acid-base regulation. See also *pH-stat acid-base regulation.*
heart function and, 15, 16t, 17
Alkalosis, prevention with CO$_2$, 24, 24–27
Alpha-stat acid-base management, anesthesia kinetics during CPB, 76–79, 77
animal studies of, in cold-blooded vertebrates, 7–8
in hibernating mammals, 11
in reptiles, 11
cerebral autoregulation during, 13, 27–29, 35
CBF and CMRO$_2$ levels and, 25–27
cortical evoked potentials and, 14
dominance of, in CPB, 4
flow-metabolism coupling and, 27–29, 35
historical background of, 3–4
intracellular neutrality and, 5–6
intracelluler-extracellular neutral pH buffering and, 6–7
ischemic heart and, 15
theory and rationale for, 4–7
Amnesia, during CPB emergence, 112
Amphibians, alpha-stat acid-base management studies in, 7–8, 11
intracellular-extracellular pH gradient in, 11
Amrinone, pharmacology of, *123*, 124
Ancrod technique, 103
Anesthesia, emergence from CPB and, 111–112, 116
impact on CPB morbidity, 92–93

Anesthesia (Continued)
  kinetics of, 69–76
    cerebral metabolism and flow, 76–79
    depth of anesthesia and, 78–79, 92–93
    drop in concentrations during CPB, 74–75
    postoperative clearance impairment and, 75
    stress response and, 79–93
    systemic flow and temperature, 79
    study design and methodology, 70t–73t, 74
  reductions in CBF and $CMRO_2$, 22–23
Animal studies of acid-base management, in cold-blooded vertebrates, 8
  in hibernating animals, 10–11
  in reptiles, 11
  in water-breathers, 8
Anticoagulants. See Heparin anticoagulation.
Antiplatelet therapy, CPB hemodynamics and, 101
Aortic pressure, CPB emergence and, 115, 115
Arterial blood pressure, post-bypass cerebral complications and, 54–57
Arterial CO_2 tension ($PaCO_2$), alpha-stat acid-base regulation and, 3
  anesthesia kinetics during CPB, 76t, 76–79, 77–78
  cerebral autoregulation during hypothermic CPB, 13
  cerebral blood flow (CBF) and, 22, 27, 56–57
  global flow-metabolism coupling and, 13
  hypothermia and CO_2, 24, 24–27
  in cold-blooded vertebrates, 7–8
  in hibernating mammals, 10
  in hypothermic patients, 8–9
  normal values for, 2
Arterial inflow line filters, 53, 69
Arterial oxygen content (C_aO_2), acid-base management and, 25–26
  cerebral blood flow (CBF) and, 22
  CPP and autoregulatory plateau in, 27–28, 28
Artificial heart, 125
Atelectasis, during CPB emergence, 113
Atheromatous debris, embolism formation and, 54
Autoregulation, anesthesia kinetics and, 77–78
  cerebral, cerebral perfusion pressure (CPP) and, 27–29
  during acid-base management of hypothermic CPB, 13
  in normal physiology, 21–22

Autoregulation (Continued)
  hypothermic alteration of, 27–28, 28, 36
  mean arterial pressure (MAP) and, 55–56
Awareness, during CPB emergence, 111–112

Balloon counterpulsation, global cerebral hypoperfusion and, 34
Barbiturates, cerebral metabolism inhibition with, 58
Bleeding (excessive), causes of, 104–105
  chest drainage criteria in, 104–105, 105t
  CPB hemodynamics and, 100–101
Blood gases, measurements of CPB emergence and, 111
  methods for, 2
  microembolism and, 34
  temperature correction of, 1–2
Blood microaggregates. See Aggregation.
Blood-plastic interface, microembolism and, 34
Bolus plus infusion techniques, anesthesia kinetics and, 74
Boundary-zone infarction, global cerebral hypoperfusion and, 33–34
  neurologic dysfunction and, 36–37
Bradycardia, CPB emergence and, 113–114
Bradykinin, postperfusion syndrome activation of, 132
Brain dysfunction. See Neurologic dysfunction.
Bronchospasm, during CPB emergence, 113
Bubble oxygenators. See also Membrane oxygenator.
  embolism generation from, 52
  microembolism and, 34
  platelet damage with, 105

CABG. See Coronary artery bypass grafting (CABG).
Calcium chloride, CPB emergence and, 117–119
Calcium entry blockers, cerebral protection from, 59–60
cAMP. See Cyclic adenosine monophosphate (cAMP).
C_aO_2. See Arterial oxygen content.
Carbon dioxide (CO_2), cerebral autoregulation and, 13
  changes in, in hypothermic patients, 8
  in hibernating mammals, 10
  pH-stat acid-base regulation and, 3

Carbon dioxide (CO_2) (Continued)
 solubility, hypothermic bypass and, 24, 24–27
 stores of, in water-breathing animals, 8
Carbon dioxide (CO_2)–bicarbonate buffer system, 6–7
Cardiac dysfunction, post-CPB factors in, 134, 137t
Cardiac electrophysiology, acid-base management and, 15, 17
Cardiac output, acid-base management hypothermic CPB and, 14–17
 CPB emergence and rate dependency, 114
 robust, impact on inflammatory response, 141–145
Cardiac rhythm, during CPB emergence, 113–114
Cardioplegia, myocardial ischemia and, 14
Cardiopulmonary bypass (CPB). See also Emergence from CPB.
 discontinuation of, 115–119
 duration of, fatal cerebral dysfunction and, 46
 global cerebral hypoperfusion and, 33–34
 morbidity and, 91–92, 92
 multivariate morbidity analysis and, 134, 138
 neuropsychologic dysfunction and, 33, 49
 reduction of inflammatory response to, 141–145
Cardiotomy suction, embolism generation from, 52–53
Carotid stenosis, post-bypass stroke incidence and, 47
Catecholamines, cerebral dysfunction and, 91–92
 CPB emergence and, 120–121
 myocardial protection with, 89–90, 90t
 stress response and, 80–82, 81–82
CBF. See Cerebral blood flow (CBF).
Cellular membrane mechanisms, intracellular-extracellular pH gradient and, 9–10
Central nervous system (CNS), post-bypass complications of cerebral protection during surgery, 57–60
 fatal cerebral damage during, 43–46
 hyperglycemia management during, 60–61
 inadequate cerebral perfusion and, 54–57, 56
 incidence of, 41–43, 42t
 macroembolization and, 53t, 53–54
 microembolization and, 52t, 52–53

Central nervous system (CNS) (Continued)
 neuropsychologic dysfunction and, 47–52
 stroke and, 44t–45t, 46–47
Cerebral blood flow (CBF). See also Cerebral oxygen consumption (CMRO₂).
 alpha-stat acid-base management and, 27–28, 35–37
 anesthesia kinetics during CPB, 22–23, 24, 76t, 76–79, 79t
 cerebral dysfunction and, 55–57
 CO_2 solubility and, 24–27
 hypothermia and, 23–24
 mean arterial pressure (MAP) and, 56, 56–57
 nonpulsatile bypass and, 31–32
 normal cerebral physiology and, 21–22
 perfusion flow rate and, 22–23, 24, 27–32
 pulsatile vs. nonpulsatile perfusion and, 31–32
Cerebral dysfunction. See Neurologic dysfunction.
Cerebral metabolic rate for glucose (CMR_{glc}), 31–32
Cerebral metabolism inhibitors, 58–59
Cerebral oxygen consumption (CMRO₂), anesthesia kinetics and, 22–23, 23, 35, 76t, 76–79, 79t
 autoregulatory plateau and, 27–28, 28
 cerebral blood flow (CBF) and, 21–22
 hypothermic inhibition of, 58–59
 nonpulsatile perfusion and, 31–32, 36
 anesthetic effects and, 22–23, 23
 cerebral perfusion pressure (CPP) and, 24–27
 CO_2 solubility in, 24–27
 flow rate in, 29–31
 hypothermia and, 23–24
 pulsatile vs. nonpulsatile, 31–32
Cerebral perfusion pressure (CPP), autoregulation during hypothermic bypass, 27–29
 in normal physiology, 22
Cerebral protection during bypass, 57–60
Cerebral steal phenomenon, anesthesia kinetics and, 78–79
Cerebral vasodilation, 78–79
Cerebrovascular disease and cerebral dysfunction post-bypass, 57
Chemical neutrality of water (pN), acid-base management and, 4, 5
 intracellular pH (pH_i) and, 6
 temperature-parallel pH in cold-blooded animals, 7–8
Chest drainage criteria, for post-CPB reentry, 104–105, 105t
Circulatory support devices, bypass emergence and, 116, 116t

Clonidine and catecholamine response, 88
Coagulation disorders, CPB hemodynamics and, 100
Cold-blooded vertebrates, alpha-stat acid-base regulation in, 7–8
Colloid osmotic sieving ratio, post-CPB, 136, 140
Communication among physicians, during bypass emergence, 115–116
Complement activation, microembolism and, 34
  pathways for, 132–133, 133
  post-CPB pulmonary dysfunction and, 137–138
  postperfusion syndrome and, 132–136
  protamine interaction with, 103, 139, 141–142
  stress response and, 80
Complement anaphylatoxins, C3a, activation by CPB, 133–134, 134–135, 138
  postperfusion syndrome and, 142–143, 143
  protamine-complement interaction and, 139, 141–142
  C4a, protamine-complement interaction and, 139, 141–142
  C5a, polymorphonuclear leukocytes and, 137–138
  post-CPB activation of, 134, 136, 138
  protamine-complement interaction and, 139, 141–142
  C5b-9, 138
Computerized infusion schemes, anesthesia kinetics and, 74, 75
Congenital heart disease (CHD), post-bypass neuropsychologic dysfunction and, 48–49
Constant alpha, defined, 7
Constant net charge, defined, 7
Coronary artery bypass grafting (CABG), catecholamine release and, 121
  fatal cerebral dysfunction and, 46
  cortisol release and, 88, 90
  neuropsychologic dysfunction and, 49, 51–52
  stroke and, 46–47
Coronary artery spasm, calcium chloride and, 118–119
Cortisol, stress response release of, 80, 82–83
  with fentanyl or alfentanil, 88, 90
Cross-clamp technique, bypass emergence and, 116
Cryoprecipitate, post-CBP hemostasis with, 105
Cyclic adenosine monophosphate (cAMP), amrinone inhibition of, 124

Defibrillator, use during CPB emergence, 113–114
Defibrinogenation with ancrod technique, 103
Delirium, post-bypass, 47–48
  preoperative conditions and, 48–49
Desmopressin, post-CPB hemostasis and, 106
Diabetics, stroke incidence in, 60
Diazepam, CBF and CMRO$_2$ levels and, 22–24, 23–24
  hypothermic-normothermic comparisons of, 23–24
  systemic flow and temperature and, 79
Digoxin, pharmacokinetics of, 75
Disseminated intravascular coagulation (DIC), 103
Dissociation constant of water (pK$_w$), pH control with, 5
Dobutamine, CPB emergence and, 120–121
Donnan equilibrium, intracellular neutrality and, 6
Dopamine, CPB emergence and, 120

EACA. See Epsilon aminocaproic acid (EACA).
Echo ultrasound, embolism detection with, 52
Echocardiography, embolism detection with, 52
Edema, post-CPB, 136, 139
Electroencephalographic (EEC) burst suppression, CBF and CMRO$_2$ levels and, 78–79
  fentanyl anesthesia and, 23–24
Emergence from CPB, amrinone and, 122, 124
  anesthetic equipment for, 111–112, 112
  cardiac rhythm and, 113–114
  discontinuing bypass during, 115–119
  inotropic agents for, 119–124
  laboratory data before, 111
  mechanical assist devices for, 125
  monitoring techniques for, 115
  preparation guidelines for, 109t, 109–110
  right ventricular failure during, 122–124
  temperature measurement and, 110–111
  vasodilators and, 121–122
  ventilation during, 113
Enflurane anesthesia, stress response and, 86, 87
Epinephrine, alpha- and beta-adrenergic agonist properties of, 88–89
  CPB emergence and, 119–121

Epinephrine (Continued)
  nitroglycerine and, 122
  plasma levels of, 87–88, 89
  stress response release of, 80–82, 81–82
Epsilon-aminocaproic acid (EACA), CPB hemodynamics and, 101, 105
Etomidate, arterial CO_2 tension ($PaCO_2$) and, 58
Excitatory amino acid (EAA), cerebral protection from, 60
Extracellular pH (pH_a), 5–11
  cardioplegia control of, 14
  in hibernating mammals, 10
  hypothermia and CO_2, 24, 24–27
  regulation of, 3
Extracellular-to-intracellular H^+ gradient, neutral pH buffering in, 6–7
Extracorporeal circulation, cerebral injury and, 51–52
  embolisms from equipment, 52
  heparin neutralization and, 101–103
Extracorporeal membrane oxygenation (ECMO), heparin anticoagulation neutralization and, 102

Factor VIII:vWF assay, CPB hemodynamics and, 100–101
Fatal cerebral damage, post-bypass, 43–46
Fentanyl, CBF and $CMRO_2$ levels and, 22–23, 23–24, 78–79
  hypothermic-normothermic comparisons of, 23–24
  CPB morbidity and, 92–93
  kinetics of, 77–78, 78
  stress response and, 87–88
  systemic flow and temperature and, 79
Fibrin microaggregates, embolism formation from, 52
Fibrinolysis, anticoagulation control and, 102–103
  postperfusion syndrome activation and, 132
Fibrinolytic therapy, CPB hemodynamics and, 101
Flow-metabolism coupling, anesthetic effects and, 22–23
  cerebral emboli and, 56
  CO_2 abolition of, 25
  intravenous and volatile anesthetics and, 35
  nonpulsatile perfusion and, 31–32
  normal cerebral physiology and, 21–22

Gallamine, pharmacokinetics of, 74
Gaseous emboli, 52–53

Global cerebral hypoperfusion, causes of, 33–34
  neurologic dysfunction and, 36–37
Global cerebral ischemia, excitatory amino acid and, 60
Gluconeogenesis, cerebral dysfunction and, 91–92
Glucose levels, cerebral dysfunction and, 91–92
  stress response and, 80, 82
Glycogenolysis, CPB emergence and, 111
Great toe temperature, CPB emergence and, 110

Hageman factor (XII) activation, 132
Halothane, systemic flow and temperature and, 79
Heart disease, neuropsychologic dysfunction post-bypass and, 48–49
Heart function. See Cardiac output.
Heart surgery, open, central nervous system complications and, 44t–45t
  preoperative factors and, 48–49
Heated humidifiers, post-bypass warming and, 111
Heating blankets, post-bypass temperature and, 111
Hematocrit, CPB emergence and, 111
Hemodilution techniques, drug pharmacokinetics and, 74–75
Hemodynamics, anesthesia kinetics and, 79
  fine tuning during emergence, 117
  hemostatic profile, CPB hemodynamics and, 100
  neurologic dysfunction and, 32
Hemostasis, during CPB, 99–106
  post-CPB, 104t, 104–106
Heparin anticoagulation, CPB hemodynamics and, 101
  hemostasis and, 99
  neutralization of, 101–103
Hibernating mammal studies, 10–11
Histidine, imidazole R-group, 6–7
Hormones, cerebral dysfunction and, 91–92, 92
  stress response and, 80–82
Human studies of alpha-stat acid-base management, 8–9
H^+/OH^- ratio, acid-base management of hypothermic CPB and, 1
  buffering systems for, 6–7
  intracellular neutrality and, 5–6
  vs. pH, 4, 5
Hyperbaric oxygen therapy, macroembolism from, 61
Hypercapnia, anesthesia kinetics and, 78–79

Hyperglycemia, management of, 60–61
  stress response and, 82
Hyperperfusion, pH-stat acid-base management and, 26–27
Hypertension, post-bypass, 122
Hyperventilation, acid-base regulation in cold-blooded animals, 8
  in hibernating mammals, 11
Hypocapnia, prevention with CO_2, 24, 24–27
Hypotension, fatal cerebral damage and, 43
  perioperative, global cerebral hypoperfusion and, 34, 36
  neurologic dysfunction and, 33
  postoperative, cerebral disorders and, 55
  protamine activation and, 103
Hypothermia, anesthesia requirements during, 75
  cerebral metabolism inhibition from, 58–59
  cerebral oxygen consumption ($CMRO_2$) and, 23–24
  enzymatic reactions and, 82
  water-breathing animals and, 8
Hypoventilation, in hibernating mammals, 11

Inflammatory response to CPB, reduction of, 141–145
Inhalation anesthetics, kinetics of, 69
  stress response and, 86–87
  systemic flow and temperature and, 79
Inotropic drugs, CPB emergence and pharmacology of, 119–124
  ventricular filling pressure and, 117–119
Insulin release, hypothermia and, 82
Intellectual/cognitive function, post-bypass, 50–52
Intra-aortic balloon pump, left ventricular dysfunction and, 125
Intracellular electrochemical neutrality, 304
Intracellular-extracellular pH gradient (pH_i-pH_a), 9–11
  in hibernating animals, 10–11
  in reptiles and amphibians, 11
Intracellular neutrality, normal cell function and, 5–6
Intracellular pH (pH_i), 5–11
  during ischemia, 15, 17
  hypothermia and brain function and, 14
  in hibernating mammals, 10
  in reptiles, 11

Intracranial pressure (ICP), cerebral perfusion pressure and, 22
  hyperbaric oxygen therapy and, 61
Intravenous anesthesia, systemic flow and temperature and, 79
Ionization constants (pK_a), imidazole protein buffer and, 7
  intracellular neutrality and, 5
Ischemia, calcium entry blockers and, 59–60
  cerebral, glucose release and, 91–92
  post-bypass stroke incidence and, 47
  protection from, 57–60
  complete global, 58–59
  myocardial, aortic cross-clamping during hypothermia and, 14
  calcium chloride and, 118–119
  ST segment elevation as sign of, 114
Ischemic tissue, acid-base regulation and, 15–17
Isoflurane anesthesia, CBF and $CMRO_2$ levels and, 23–24, 35, 78–79
  cerebral metabolism inhibition and, 58
  cortisol response and, 86, 88
  emergence from CPB and, 112
  systemic flow and temperature and, 79
  washout curves in, 112
Isoproterenol, CPB emergence and, 120–121
  right ventricular failure and, 123–124

Jugular venous oxygen saturation ($S_{jv}O_2$), hypothermic alpha-stat CBP and, 28–29

Kallikrein system, postperfusion syndrome activation, 132

Lactate dehydrogenase, inhibition in hibernating mammals, 10
Left ventricular dysfunction, epinephrine action and, 119–121
  intraluminal defects, embolism formation and, 54
  thrombi, post-bypass stroke incidence and, 47
Leukocyte aggregates, embolism formation from, 52
Lidocaine, cerebral protection from, 60
  pharmacokinetics of, 74–75, 75
Lipid membranes, acid-base management and, 8
Lipid solubility, drug pharmacokinetics and, 74–75
Lipoprotein denaturation, fat microembolism and, 34

Low cardiac output state, global cerebral hypoperfusion and, 34, 36

Low flow/low pressure bypass technique, cerebral disorders and, 55

"Luxury perfusion" concept, acid-base management of hypothermia and, 25–26

Lympha-plasma protein ratio, post-CPB, 136, 140

Macroembolism, 35
 causes of, 53t
 fatal cerebral damage and, 43–46
 morbidity from, 36
 neurologic dysfunction and, 32

Mean arterial pressure (MAP), acid-base management and, 25–26, 26
 autoregulation and, 27–29
 cerebral blood flow (CBF) and, 56, 56–57
 cerebral perfusion pressure and, 22
 global cerebral hypoperfusion and, 34
 inadequate cerebral perfusion and, 54–57
 jugular venous O_2 saturation $(S_{jv}O_2)$ and, 28–29, 30
 neurologic dysfunction and, 33
 perfusion flow rate and, 36

Membrane oxygenator. See also Bubble oxygenators.
 cerebral blood flow (CBF) and, 31–32
 inflammatory response and, 143, 144
 platelet damage with, 105

Metabolism, depression of, in hibernating mammals, 10–11

Microembolism, cerebral damage and, 52–53
 neurologic dysfunction and, 36–37
 post-bypass, 34
 types of, 52t

Microvascular permeability, alterations in post-CPB, 136, 139

Midazolam, arterial CO_2 tension $(PaCO_2)$ and, 58
 pharmacokinetics of, 75

"Milieu interieur," 5

Multiple-valve procedures, neuropsychologic dysfunction and, 49

Muscle glycolysis, in hibernating mammals, 10

Myocardial preservation, bypass emergence and, 116

Nasopharyngeal temperature, anesthesia kinetics during CPB, 76t, 76
 cerebral blood flow (CBF) and, 27, 56–57
 emergence from CBF, 110

Neurologic dysfunction. See also Central nervous system (CNS).
 acid-base management of hypothermic CPB and, 12–14
 causes of, 33–37
 clinical correlates, 32–33, 33t
 embolism and, 34–35, 91–93
 factors in, 32–33, 33t
 global cerebral hypoperfusion and, 33–34
 manifestations and incidence of, 32, 32t
 preexisting deficits and, 33

Neuropsychologic dysfunction, intellectual/cognitive changes in, 50–52
 perioperative factors and, 49
 post-bypass delirium and organic brain syndrome and, 47–48
 postoperative factors and, 49–50
 preoperative factors and, 48–49

Nicardipine, cerebral protection from, 59–60

Nimodipine, cerebral protection from, 59–60

Nitroglycerine, post-bypass hypertension and, 122

Nitroprusside. See also Sodium nitroprusside.
 vasodilation induction and, 110–111

Nomograms, body temperature measurement with, 2
 development of, 3

Nonpulsatile bypass, anesthesia kinetics during, 77
 cerebral oxygen consumption $(CMRO_2)$ levels and, 36
 suboptimal oxygen delivery during, 31–32

Norepinephrine, alpha- and beta-adrenergic agonist properties of, 88–89
 CPB emergence and, 120–121
 sparing effect of, 86
 stress response release of, 80–82, 81–82

Norepinephrine-mediated nonshivering thermogenesis, 10

Open heart surgery, central nervous system complications and, 44t–45t
 preoperative factors and, 48–49

Open-ventricle procedures, macroembolism and, 35, 36
 neurologic dysfunction post-bypass, 33

Opioids, stress response and, 86–87, 89

Optical fluorescence bypass methods, blood gas measurement with, 2

Organic brain syndrome, post-bypass, 47–48
 preoperative conditions and, 48–49

Pacemaker, CPB emergence and, 113–114
PaCO₂. See *Arterial CO₂ tension (PaCO₂)*.
Parieto-occipital "boundary zone," global
   cerebral hypoperfusion and, 33–34
Patient history, CPB hemodynamics and,
   100–101
Perfusion flow rate (Q). See also *Postper-*
   fusion syndrome.
  cerebral blood flow and, 29–31
   anesthetics and, 22–23, *23–24*
   CO₂ solubility and, 24–27
   cerebral oxygen consumption
    (CMRO₂) and, 22–32
   cerebral perfusion pressure (CPP)
    and, 27–31
   hypothermia and, 23–24
   metabolism and, 21
   pulsatile vs. nonpulsatile perfusion
    and, 31–32
  cerebral damage from, 54–57
  global cerebral hypoperfusion and, 34
  jugular venous O₂ saturation (S$_{jv}$O₂)
   and, 28–29
  mean arterial pressure (MAP) and, 36
  neurologic dysfunction and, 32
  optimal rates for, 57
  post-bypass temperature drop and,
   110–111
  pulsatile vs. nonpulsatile perfusion
   and, 31–32
Peripheral circulation, CPB emergence
   and, 121–122
pH, arterial, in cold-blooded vertebrates,
   7–8
  maintenance in hypothermic patients, 8–9
  extracellular. See *Extracellular pH*
   (pH$_a$).
  vs. H⁺/OH⁻ ratio, *4, 5*
  intracellular. See *Intracellular pH*
   (pH$_i$).
  normal values for, 2
  temperature changes and, in humans,
   8–9
  neutrality of, 6–7
pH-stat acid-base management, cerebral
   autoregulation and, 13–14
  CBF and CMRO₂ levels and, 25–27
  historical background of, 2–3
  in hibernating mammals, 10–11
  ischemic heart and, 15
  MAP and, 25–27, *26*
  normal vs. corrected pH-PaCO₂ values
   and, 3
  pressure-dependent cerebral hyperperfusion and, 35
  in reptiles, 11
pH$_a$. See *Extracellular pH (pH$_a$)*.

Phentolamine, post-bypass hypertension
   and, 122
Phenylephrine, hypothermic bypass and,
   89
Phenytoin, cerebral protection from, 60
Phosphodiesterase, amrinone inhibition
   of, 124
Phosphofructokinase activity, inhibition
   in hibernating mammals, 10
Phospholipid composition, acid-base
   management and, 8
Plaque debris, embolism formation from,
   53–54
Plasma catecholamines, stress response
   and, 81–82
Plasma proteins, and post-CPB permeability, 136, *140*
Platelet activation, microembolism and,
   34
  inflammatory response and, 143, 145
  in pediatric patients, 85
  thromboxane release and, 85–86
Platelet aggregates, embolism formation
   from, 52
Platelet function, during post-CPB, 104–
   105
Platelet transfusion, post-CPB bleeding
   and, 105
Poikilotherms, alpha-stat acid-base regulation in, 7–8
Polymorphonuclear leukocytes, post-CPB
   binding to C5a, 137–138
Postcardiotomy delirium, 48
Postperfusion syndrome, complement activation and, 132–133, *133*
  defined, 131
  inflammatory response during CPB,
   141–145
  microvascular permeability and, 136,
   139
  schematic of, *132*
Preoperative evaluation, hemodynamics
   during CPB and, 100–101
Pressure transducers, CPB emergence
   and, 115
Properdin complement pathway, CPB activation of, 134
  inflammatory response and, 143, 145
  pulmonary dysfunction and, 138
  schematic of, 133, *133*
Prostacyclin, autoregulatory thresholds
   during CPB, 28–29, *30*
  low arterial pressure and, 55
  stress response release of, 83–86, *84*
Prostaglandin E₁, right ventricular failure
   and, 123
Prostaglandins, stress response release of,
   80, 83

Protamine activation, complement interaction with, 139, 141–142
heparin anticoagulation neutralization and, 101–102
side effects of, 103
Protein structure and function, acid-base regulation of, 4–5
Protein buffers, neutral pH and, 6–7
Pulmonary compliance, during CPB emergence, 113
Pulmonary dysfunction, complement activation and, 137–138
post-CPB factors, 134, 137t
Pulsatile flow, post-bypass temperature and, 110–111
postperfusion syndrome and, 142
Pump oxygenator. See also *Membrane oxygenator.*
anesthesia kinetics and, 69
embolism generation with, 52

Receptor antagonists, cerebral protection from, 60
Rectal temperature, CPB emergence and, 110
Renal dysfunction, duration of CPB and, 75
post-CPB factors, 134, 137t
Reptiles, intracellular-extracellular pH gradient in, 11
Right hemispheric stroke, macroembolism and, 35
Right ventricular failure, during bypass emergence, 122–124

Selective membrane permeability, intracellular-extracellular pH gradient and, 9–10
Silicon emboli, 52
Sinus rhythm, CPB emergence and, 113–114
Sinus tachycardia, CPB emergence and, 114
Socioeconomic levels, neuropsychologic dysfunction post-bypass and, 48
Sodium nitroprusside (SNP), cerebral blood flow (CBF) and, 29
cyanide toxicity of, 122
Somatosensory-evoked potentials (SEPS), hypothermic circulatory arrest and, 14
perfusion flow rate and, 30–31
prostacyclin-induced hypotension, 29
ST segment evaluation, CPB emergence, 114

Starling mechanism, CPB emergence, 117
Stenosis, cerebral shunting during CPB, 78–79
Streptokinase, CPB hemodynamics and, 101
Stress response, anesthesia kinetics and, 79–88
CPB morbidity and, 92–93
organs and sites of, *80*
Stroke, post-bypass, 44t–45t, 46–47
Study design and methodology, anesthesia kinetics and, 69–74
neuropsychologic testing post-bypass and, 50–52
post-bypass complications data and, 43
stroke data and, 46–47
Sufentanil, stress response and, 86
Surgical repair quality, bypass emergence and, 116
Sympathetic nervous system, response to CPB, 80
Sympathoadrenal response, 80

Tachycardia, CPB emergence and, 114
Temperature, "afterdrop" during CPB emergence, 110
anesthesia kinetics and, 78, 79
blood gas correction with, 1–2
cerebral autoregulation during hypothermic CPB, 13
dissociation constant of water (pK$_w$) and, 5
emergence from CPB and, 110–111
Terminal complement complex (TCC), levels during CPB, 134, *135*
Thiopental, CBF and CMRO$_2$ levels and, 23–24 35, 78–79
neuropsychologic dysfunction and, 59
pharmacokinetics of, 74–75
Thrombi release, embolism formation and, 54
Thrombocytopenia, heparin-induced, 101
Thromboxane, stress response release and, *83*, 83–86
synthesis in pediatric patients and, 85, *85*
Tissue oxygenation, hyperbaric oxygen therapy and, 61
Transesophageal echo, for CPB emergence, 117
Transluminal coronary artery angioplasty, CPB hemodynamics and, 101
Transpulmonary leukocyte sequestration, 137–138
membrane oxygenator and, 143, *144*
d-Tubocurarine, pharmacokinetics of, 74

Urine temperature, CPB emergence and, 110

Valsalva maneuver, during CPB emergence, 113
Valve replacement, embolism formation and, 54
Vasoactive peptides, cerebral dysfunction and, 91–92, 92
Vasodilation, CPB emergence and, 121–122
  post-bypass temperature drop and, 110–111
  reassessment during CPB emergence, 112
Venous reservoir, anesthesia kinetics and, 69

Ventilation, acid-base regulation in cold-blooded animals, 8
  during CPB emergence, 113
Ventricular assist devices, 125
Ventricular dysfunction, preoperative, bypass emergence and, 116
Ventricular filling pressure, CPB emergence and, 117–118
Ventricullar fibrillation, CPB emergence and, 113–114
Volatile anesthetics, CPB emergence and, 112
  flow-metabolism coupling and, 23–24

Whole blood therapy, post-CPB hemostasis and, 106
"Whole body inflammatory response," 131–132